THE ULTIMATE
INTERVIEW
BIOLOGICAL SCIENCES

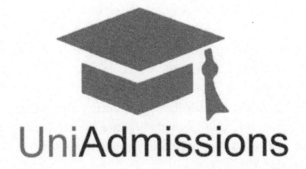

UniAdmissions

Published by *RAR Medical Services Limited*

www.uniadmissions.co.uk

info@uniadmissions.co.uk

Tel: +44 (0) 208 068 0438

THE ULTIMATE OXBRIDGE INTERVIEW GUIDE BIOLOGICAL SCIENCES

CHLOE BOWMAN

CAROLINA VALENSISE

MATTHEW FOX

DR. ROHAN AGARWAL

EDITED BY
DR. RANJNA GARG

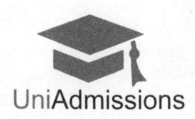

UniAdmissions

About the Authors

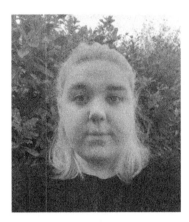

Chloe graduated with an **MEng in Engineering Science** from **Keble College, Oxford** in 2019. During her time at Oxford she researched the use of Carbon Nano Tubes in a joint project with a team at the Large Hadron Collider at CERN. She was also awarded several national engineering scholarships sponsored by the Institute of Mechanical Engineers, Institute of Engineering Technology, and Jaguar Land Rover among others.

Chloe has since begun to study for a second Master's degree in Managing Technological Development, as well as having articles published in national and online press such as The Huffington Post. Since university, Chloe works as a tutor and educational consultant, specialising in supporting students applying to Science, Technology, Engineering, and Maths degrees at Oxford and Cambridge. Outside science and education, Chloe enjoys baking and tending to her aquaponics system!

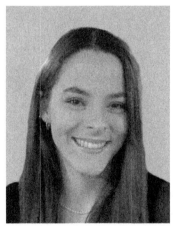

Carolina is a fifth-year medical student at the **University of Oxford**. After achieving a BA in Medical Sciences in 2020 she is now halfway through her clinical training, having particular academic interests in acute care, paediatrics and holistic medicine. She is the current President of Osler House, the common room representing Oxford's clinical medical students nationally on academic and non-academic matters.

Carolina is additionally a keen teacher and passionate about medical education, leading a widening participation tutoring initiative for prospective medical students from underrepresented backgrounds.

Matthew is a third-year chemistry student at the University of Cambridge. His current specialty is in synthetic chemistry and the manufacturing of complex chemicals. He plans to develop this into postgraduate study developing an even greater expertise in organic chemistry, which not only will support his career as a chemist but allow him to provide a broad base of chemistry tutoring and education. In his spare time, he plays squash on his college team and enjoys cycling.

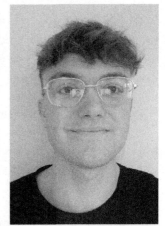

Rohan is the **Director of Operations** at *UniAdmissions* and is responsible for its technical and commercial arms. He graduated from Gonville and Caius College, Cambridge and is a fully qualified doctor. Over the last five years, he has tutored hundreds of successful Oxbridge and Medical applicants. He has also authored ten books on admissions tests and interviews.

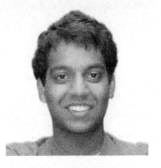

Rohan has taught physiology to undergraduates and interviewed medical school applicants for Cambridge. He has published research on bone physiology and writes education articles for the Independent and Huffington Post. In his spare time, Rohan enjoys playing the piano and table tennis.

Preface

Oxbridge interviews are frequently the source of intriguing stories. You'll frequently hear tales of students who were asked seemingly obscure questions e.g. "Why do we have two nostrils but only one mouth?", or impossibly difficult ones e.g. "How many grains of sand are there in the world?"

If taken in context, both of these are very fair Oxbridge interview questions. The first would naturally lead to a discussion concerning the evolution of sensory organs and the pros/cons of having multiple mouths e.g. reduced risk of infections vs. inability to eat and speak simultaneously etc.

The latter question would test a candidate's ability to breakdown an initially very large problem into more bite-sized chunks in order to manage it e.g. surface area of the Earth, percentage of the Earth covered by land, percentage of land covered by sand, average depth of sand and so on.

Oxbridge interviews are not about testing your knowledge. Instead, they are about testing what you can do with the knowledge you already possess. Remember, once you're at university, you will rapidly assimilate a great deal of new information (so much so that you will start to wonder what all the fuss A-levels were about).

This is the main reason why it's not particularly useful for interviewers to ask purely knowledge-based questions e.g. "What is the normal plasma concentration of magnesium?". Knowledge of isolated facts is neither necessary nor sufficient for a successful Oxbridge interview. Instead, it is the application of some basic facts to novel situations that is the hallmark of success.

To help demonstrate what we mean a little further, Rohan is going to talk through his interview experiences.

INTERVIEW ONE

This was my first science interview and the interviewer was delighted when he found out I studied physics at A2. His opening question was "What have you read recently?" I explained I'd been reading about the new drug Rosuvastatin – a statin that was being recommended for everyone above a certain age (regardless of their actual cholesterol levels). The follow-up questions were what you would expect e.g. "How do statins work?" (Ensure you know the basics of any topic that you voluntarily bring up), "What are the risks/benefits of giving them to everyone?"

This led to a discussion on how I would convince someone that this drug was useful for them, followed by how I would convince someone that blue light was more damaging than red. I struggled with this for a while, bouncing ideas back and forth (with each of them sequentially shot down) until I finally stumbled onto Einstein's $E=hf$. This led to a discussion about why the sky is blue and sunsets can be a myriad of colours. All of this culminated in the classic- "What colour is the Sun in reality?" (Hint: It's not yellow, orange or red!) This is the question that tabloids would take out of context to make the interview seem like an array of bizarre questions when in fact this was perfectly reasonable giving the preceding questions.

This interview serves as a perfect example of a non-scripted interview, i.e. one where the interviewer was happy to bounce ideas between us and forced me to think about concepts in ways I never had. I'm certain that if I had offered a different answer to the initial question about my reading, the discussion would have gone along a significantly different route.

INTERVIEW TWO

My second interview was more scripted – the interviewer had a pre-set agenda with corresponding questions that he wanted to discuss. Given that this person is known to ask the same interview questions annually, I've refrained from including specifics in order to not spoil the plot for everyone and to unfairly put future applicants at an advantage (or disadvantage!).

After going through my BMAT essay very briefly, he asked me to draw a graph on his whiteboard. This was no easy task. I spent fifteen minutes struggling with this graph due to its unusual axis. Like many candidates, I made the mistake of learning about excessively complex topics like the Complement Membrane attack complex and ignored many of the core A-level topics like human physiology. This meant that I wasn't completely sure about a basic fact that was required for the graph. This was a tough interview and at the end of it, I was certain I had flunked it. This was compounded by the fact that other candidates were bragging about how they had got the correct graph in only thirty seconds.

When you're in the waiting room with the other candidates, it may appear that many of them are far smarter than you and know a lot more. Again, remember that the entire point of an interview is to assess your ability to apply knowledge.

People get nervous and lose confidence whilst waiting for interviews. One of the ways they try to feel more secure is by exerting their intellectual superiority. In this example (although there were some exceptions), the students who tended to arrive at the answer very quickly were unsuccessful. This is likely because they had previous knowledge of the question from their school/extra reading. Although this allowed them to get the correct answer quickly, they were unable to clearly *show their thinking*, i.e. they knew the topic but didn't understand it.

LEARNING POINTS

As you can see, I made lots of errors in my interview preparation. Please learn from them. Good students learn from their mistakes but great students learn from others' mistakes.

1. Don't be put off by what other candidates say in the waiting room. Focus on yourself – you are all that matters. If you want to be in the zone, then I would recommend taking some headphones and your favourite music.
2. Don't read up on multiple advanced topics in depth. Choose one topic and know it well. Focus the rest of your time on your core A-level syllabus. A medic is not expected to know about the features of Transverse Myelitis, but you will be expected to be able to rattle off a list of 10 cellular organelles.
3. Don't worry about being asked seemingly irrelevant questions that you'll often hear in the media. These are taken out of context. Focus on being able to answer the common questions e.g. "Why this university?" etc.
4. Don't lose heart if your interviews appear to have gone poorly. If anything, this can actually be a good sign as it shows that the interviewer pushed you to your limits rather than giving up on you as you clearly weren't Oxbridge material.
5. Don't give up. When you're presented with complex scenarios, go back to the absolute basics and try to work things out using first principles. By doing this and thinking out loud, you allow the interviewer to see your logical train of thought so that they can help you when you become stuck.

Good Luck!

Dr Rohan Agarwal

CONTENTS

THE BASICS

WHAT IS AN OXBRIDGE INTERVIEW?

An interview is a personal session with one or two members of academic staff from Oxford or Cambridge, usually lasting anywhere between 20 and 50 minutes. The interviewers will ask questions and guide the applicant to an answer. The answers usually require a large degree of creative and critical thought, as well as a good attitude and a sound foundation of subject-specific knowledge.

WHY IS THERE AN INTERVIEW?

Most of the applicants to Oxbridge will have outstanding grades, predicted exam results, sample course work and personal statements. Interviews are used to help determine which applicants are best-suited for Oxbridge. During the interview, each applicant has a unique chance to demonstrate their creativity and critical thinking abilities - skills that Oxford and Cambridge consider vital for successful students.

WHO GETS AN INTERVIEW?

At Cambridge, any applicant who might have a chance at being accepted to study will be called for interview. This corresponds to approximately 90% of applicants. At Oxford, odds of getting interviewed are lower, due to a mixture of factors including applicant numbers and selection criteria, and you're on average about 40% likely to be invited to interview. No one is offered a place to study without attending an interview.

WHO ARE THE INTERVIEWERS?

The interviews are conducted by a senior member of staff for the subject you've applied to; usually this person is the Director of Studies for that subject. There may often be a second interviewer who takes notes on the applicant or also asks questions. Interviewers describe this experience as just as nerve-wracking for them as for the applicants, as they are responsible for choosing the right students for Oxford and Cambridge.

WHEN IS THE INTERVIEW?

Interviews are held in the beginning of December and some applicants may be invited back in January for a second round of interviews at another college. There are usually multiple interviews on the same day, either for different subjects or at different colleges. You will normally be given 2 weeks' notice before your interview- so you should hear back by late November, but it is useful to begin preparing for the interview before you're officially invited.

WHERE IS THE INTERVIEW?

The interviews are held in Oxford and Cambridge at the college you applied to. Oxford applicants may have additional interviews at another college than the one applied to. Cambridge applicants may get 'pooled' – be required to have another set of interviews in January at a different college. If you are travelling from far away, most Oxbridge colleges will provide you free accommodation and food for the duration of your stay if you wish to arrive the night before your interview.

Very rarely, interviews can be held via Skype at an exam centre- this normally only applies to international students or for UK students in extreme circumstances. During a pandemic, interviews are usually held on Microsoft Teams.

Finally, work your way through the past interview questions – remember, you are not expected to know the answers to them, and they have been included here so that you can start to appreciate the style of questions that you may get asked. It is not a test of what you know – but what you can do with what you already know.

OXBRIDGE TUTORIALS & SUPERVISIONS

Hopefully, by this point, you're familiar with the unique Oxbridge teaching system. Students on the same course will have lectures and practicals together. These are supplemented by college-based tutorials/supervisions. A tutorial/supervision is an individual or small group session with an academic to discuss ideas, ask questions, and receive feedback on your assignments. During the tutorial/supervision, you will be pushed to think critically about the material from the course in novel and innovative ways. To get the most out of Oxbridge, you need to be able to work in this setting and take criticism with a positive and constructive attitude.

The interviews are made to be model tutorials/supervisions, with an academic questioning an applicant and seeing if they can learn, problem-solve, demonstrate motivation for their subject. It is by considering this ultimate goal of the interview that you can start to understand how to present and prepare yourself for the Oxbridge interview process.

WHAT ARE INTERVIEWERS LOOKING FOR?

There are several qualities an interviewer is looking for the applicant to demonstrate during the interview. While an applicant may think the most 'obvious' thing interviewers are looking for is excellent factual knowledge, this is already displayed through exam results. Whilst having an excellent depth of knowledge may help you perform better during an interview, you're unlikely to be chosen based solely on your knowledge. The main thing an interviewer is looking for is for the applicant to demonstrate critical thought, excellent problem-solving skills and intellectual flexibility, as well as motivation for the subject and suitability for small group teaching. It is also important for them to see that the applicant is willing to persevere with a challenging problem even if the answer is not immediately apparent.

HOW TO COMMUNICATE ANSWERS

The most important thing to do when communicating your answers is to think out loud. This will allow the interviewer to understand your thought processes. They will then be able to help you out if you get stuck. You should never give up on a question; show that you won't be perturbed at the first sign of hardship as a student, and remain positive and demonstrate your engagement with the material. Interviewers enjoy teaching and working with students who are as enthusiastic about their subject as they are.

Try to keep the flow of conversation going between you and your interviewer so that you can engage with each other throughout the entire interview. The best way to do this is to just keep talking about what you are thinking. It is okay to take a moment when confronted with a difficult question or plan your approach, but ensure you let the interviewer know this by saying, "I'm going to think about this for a moment". Don't take too long - if you are finding the problems difficult, the interviewers will guide and prompt you to keep you moving forward. They can only do this if they know you're stuck!

The questions that you'll be asked are designed to be difficult, so don't panic up when you don't immediately know the answer. Tell the interviewer what you do know, offer some ideas, talk about ways you've worked through a similar problem that might apply here. If you've never heard anything like the question asked before, say that to the interviewer, "I've never seen anything like this before" or "We haven't covered this yet at school", but don't use that as an excuse to quit. This is your chance to show that you are eager to engage with new ideas, so finish with "But let's see if I can figure it out!" or "But I'm keen to try something new!". There are many times at Oxbridge when students are in this situation during tutorials/supervisors and you need to show that you can persevere in the face of difficulty (and stay positive and pleasant to work with while doing so).

TYPES OF INTERVIEWS

There are, at Cambridge and for some Oxford subjects, several different types of interview that you can be called for. Every applicant will have at least one subject interview. Applicants to some courses may also have a general interview, especially if they are applying for an arts subject. Either way, you will be asked questions that touch on the course you are applying to study. It may be useful to look at your interviewers' teaching backgrounds and published work as this could potentially shed some light on the topics they might choose to discuss in an interview. However, there is absolutely no need to know the intricacies of their research so don't get bogged down in it. Interviews tend to open with easier and more general questions and become more detailed and complicated as you are pushed to explore topics in greater depth.

USING THE PRACTICE QUESTIONS

This book contains over 900 practice interview questions. They are all actual questions that successful Oxbridge applicants were asked in their interview. However, it is important you take these with a pinch of salt.

They are taken out of context and only included to give you a flavour of the style and difficulty of real Oxbridge interview questions. Don't fall into the trap of thinking that your interview will consist of a series of disconnected and highly specific knowledge-based questions.

OXBRIDGE INTERVIEWS ARE **NOT** ABOUT YOUR KNOWLEDGE

THEY ARE ABOUT WHAT YOU CAN DO WITH THE KNOWLEDGE YOU ALREADY POSSESS

Thus, it does little benefit to rote learn answers to all the practice questions in this book as they are unlikely to be repeated. Instead, follow our top tips, take inspiration from the worked answers and put in some hard work – you'll be sure to perform well on the day.

GENERAL INTERVIEWS

A general interview is a get-to-know-you session with senior admissions tutors. This is your chance to demonstrate a passion for Oxbridge; that you have understood the Oxbridge system, have a genuine interest in being a student, and could contribute to Oxbridge if you were admitted. These are more common for arts and humanities applicants, but all applicants should nevertheless be prepared for a general interview.

- This will be less specific than the subject interview. The interviewers will focus more on your personal statement, any essays you may have submitted or have completed on the day of the interview and may discuss your SAQ form if you are applying to Cambridge.
- One of the interviewers may not be a specialist in the subject you've applied for. Don't be put off by this – you aren't expected to have any knowledge of their subject.
- Ensure that you have read your personal statement and any books/journals that you've claimed to have read in your application. You will seem unenthusiastic and dishonest if you can't answer questions regarding topics and activities that you claim to know about. Remember that it is much better to show a good understanding of a few texts than to list lots of texts that you haven't properly read.
- Read and re-read the essays you have submitted (if you have done). Be prepared to expand on the ideas you have explored in them. Remember that the interviewers may criticise what you've argued in your submitted essays. If you believe in it, then defend your view but don't be stubborn.
- You will normally be asked if you have any questions at the end of the interview. Avoid saying things like, "How did I do?" – Instead use this as an opportunity to show the interviewers the type of person you are e.g. "How many books can I borrow from the library at one time?"

WHAT TYPE OF QUESTIONS MIGHT BE ASKED?

The three main questions that are likely to come up in an Oxbridge interview are:

- Why this university?
- Why this subject?
- Why this college?

You may also get asked more specific questions about the teaching system or about your future career aspirations. This will also be the time for discussing any extenuating circumstances for poor exam results and similar considerations.

To do well in a general interview, your answers should show that you understand the Oxbridge system and that you have strong reasons for applying there. Thus, it is essential that you prepare detailed answers to the common questions above so that you aren't caught off guard. In addition, you should create a list of questions that could potentially be asked based on your personal statement or any submitted work.

WORKED QUESTIONS

Below are a few examples of how to start breaking down general interview questions- complete with model answers.

Q1: How did you choose which college to apply for?

This question is a good opportunity to tell the interviewer about yourself, your hobbies, motivations, and any interesting projects you have undertaken. You can demonstrate that you have read about the College thoroughly and you know what differentiates your College from the others. The decisive factors can include a great variety of different things from history, alumni, location in the city, community, sports clubs, societies, any positive personal experiences from Open Day and notable scholars.

This is a warm up question – an ice-breaker – so just be natural and give an honest answer. You may not want to say things like, "I like the statues in the garden". The more comprehensive your answer is, the better.

Good Applicant: I chose which college to apply for based on a number of factors that were important to me. First of all, I needed to consider how many other students at my college would be studying the same subject as me; this was important to me as I want to be able to engage in conversation about my subject with my peers. Secondly, I considered the location of the college as I wanted to ensure I had easy access to the faculty library and lecture theatres. Thirdly, I am a keen tennis player and so looked for a college with a very active tennis society. Finally, I wanted to ensure that the college I chose would feel right for me and so I looked around several Cambridge colleges before coming to my conclusion.

This response is broken down into a set of logical and yet personal reasons. **There is no right answer to this question** and the factors which influence this decision are likely to be unique for each individual. However, each college is unique and therefore the interviewer wants to know what influenced your decision. Therefore, **it's essential that you know what makes your college special** and separates it from the others. Even more importantly, you should know what the significance of that will be for you. For example, if a college has a large number of mathematicians, you may want to say that, by attending that college, it would allow you to discuss your subject with a greater number of people than otherwise.

A **poor applicant** may respond with a noncommittal shrug or an answer such as, "my brother went there". The interviewers want to see that you have researched the university and although the reason for choosing a college won't determine whether or not you get into the university, a lack of passion and interest in the college will greatly influence how you are perceived by the interviewers.

Q2: Why have you chosen to apply to study at 'Oxbridge', rather than another Russell Group university?

This is a very broad question and one which is simply designed to draw out the motives and thinking behind your application, as well as giving you an opportunity to speak freely about yourself.

A **good applicant** would seek to address this question in two parts, the first addressing the key features of Oxbridge for their course and the second emphasising their own personality traits and interests which make them most suited to the Oxbridge system.

It is useful to start off by talking about the supervision/tutorial system and why this method of very small group teaching is beneficial for studying your subject, both for the discussion of essay work and, more crucially, for developing a comprehensive understanding of your subject. You might also like to draw upon the key features of the course at Oxford and Cambridge that distinguish it from courses at other universities.

When talking about yourself, a good answer could take almost any route, though it is always productive to talk about which parts of your subject interest you, why this is the case, and how this ties in with the course at Oxford/Cambridge. You might also mention how the Oxbridge ethos suits your personality, e.g. how hard work and high achievement are important to you and you want to study your chosen subject in real depth, rather than a more superficial course elsewhere.

A **poor applicant** would likely demonstrate little or no knowledge of their course at Oxford/Cambridge and volunteer little information about why studying at Oxbridge would be good for them or why they would be suited to it. It's important to focus on your interests and abilities rather than implying that you applied because Oxbridge is the biggest name or because your family or school had expected you to do so.

Q3: What do you think you can bring to the college experience?

This is a common question at general interviews and **you need to show that you would be a good fit for the College** and that you are also really motivated because you have researched the college's facilities, notable fellows and alumni, societies and sports clubs etc. You can mention that you have looked at the website, talked to alumni and current students.

This question also gives the interviewer an excellent opportunity to learn about your personality, hobbies and motivations. Try to avoid listing one thing after the other for 5 minutes. Instead, you should try to give a balanced answer in terms of talking about the College and yourself. You should talk about your skills and give examples when you had to work in a team, deliver on strict deadlines, show strong time-management skills etc. You should also give a few examples from your previous studies, competitions or extracurricular activities (including sports and music).

Q4: Tell me about a recent news article not related to your subject that has interested you.

This can be absolutely anything and your interviewers just want to see that **you are aware of the world in which you live** and have a life outside of your subject. You could pick an interesting topic ahead of time and cultivate an opinion which could spark a lively discussion.

Q5: Which three famous people would you most like to be stuck on a desert island with?

This is a personal question that might be used by your interviewers as an 'ice-breaker' – you can say absolutely anyone but try to have a good justification (and avoid being melodramatic). This is a really **good chance to show your personality and sense of humour**. This is also a good question to ease you into the flow of the interview and make you feel more comfortable.

Q6: Do you think you're 'clever'?

Don't let this one faze you! Your interviewers are not being glib but instead want to see how you cope with questions you may not have anticipated. You could discuss different forms of intelligence, e.g. emotional vs. intellectual, perhaps concluding that you are stronger in one over the other.

Q7: What experiences do you have which suggest to you that you'll cope well with the pressures of Oxbridge?

The **interviewers want to hear that you know what you're signing up** to and that you are capable of dealing with stress. If you have any experience of dealing with pressure or meeting strict deadlines, this would be a good opportunity to talk about them. Otherwise, mention your time management skills and your ability to prioritise workloads. You could also mention how you deal with stress, e.g. do you like running? Yoga? Piano? Etc.

Q8: Why are you in this room?

There are hundreds of potential responses to this type of question, and the interviewer will see this as a chance to get to know your personality and how you react to unusual situations.

Firstly, **take the question seriously**, even if it strikes you as funny or bizarre. A good response may begin with: "There are many reasons why I am in this room. There are lots of smaller events and causes that have led up to me being in this room". You might choose to discuss your desire to attend Oxbridge, the fact that you have travelled to the college to take your interview. You might choose to discuss the interviewer or college's taste and budget when it came to allocating rooms for interviews, as that determined why and how you have come to be sitting in that room, rather than anywhere else.

A weak response to this type of question would be to dismiss it as silly or irrelevant.

Q9: Let's say you're hosting a small private party, and you have a magical invitation that will summon anyone from time and space to your dining table. Who's name do you write on the invitation?

This is a fairly straightforward question to get in a general interview, so use it to show your personality and originality, and to talk about something you are passionate about.

If you are asked a question like this, give an answer that is relevant to your application. This is not the time to start talking about how you are a huge fan of Beyonce and would just love to have dinner together! You should also avoid generic answers like "God".

If you would love to meet Barack Obama and know more about him, consider what that would be like. Would he be at liberty to answer your questions? Might you not get more information from one of his aides or from a close friend, rather than the man himself? As this is a simple question, try to unpick it and answer it in a sophisticated way, rather than just stating the obvious.

Q10: What was the most recent film you watched?

This question seems simple and appears to require a relatively short answer. However, a good candidate will use a simple question such as this as an opportunity to speak in more depth and **raise new and interesting topics of conversation**: "What I find particularly interesting about this film was... It reminded me of... In relation to other works of this period/historical context, I found this particular scene very interesting as it mirrored/contrasted with my previous conceptions of this era as seen in other works, for example... I am now curious to find out more about... This film made me think about...etc."

Whilst it is extremely important to respond accurately to the questions posed by the interviewer, do not be afraid to **take the conversation in the direction led by your personal interests**. This sort of initiative will be encouraged.

Q11: How do you think the university will evaluate whether or not you have done well at the end of your degree, do you think that this manner of assessment is fair?

This question invites you to show your potential and how diverse your interests are. There are three aspects of this question that you should consider in order to give a complete answer: "end of your degree", "evaluate" and "done well". You may want to discuss your hobbies and interests and potential achievements regarding various aspects of university life including academia, sports, student societies, jobs, volunteering etc.

Then you may want to enter into a discussion about whether there is any fair measure of success. How could you possibly compare sporting excellence to volunteering? Is it better to be a specialist or a generalist? This ultimately comes down to your personal motivation and interests as you might be very focused on your studies or other activities (e.g. sports, music). Thus, multiple things would contribute to your success at university and your degree is only likely to be one way to measure this. Finally, it might be a great closing line to mention that getting your degree might not be the end of your time here.

Q12: Tell me why you think people should go to university.

This sounds like a very general question at first but it is, in fact, about your personal motivations to go to university. You don't need to enter into a discussion about what universities are designed for or any educational policy issues as the interviewer is unlikely to drive the discussion towards this in a general interview.

The best strategy is to **discuss your motivations**- this could include a broad range of different things from interest in a certain field, inspiring and diverse environments, academic excellence, opening up of more opportunities in the future and buying time to find out more about yourself etc. As it is very easy to give an unfocused answer, you should limit yourself to a few factors. You can also comment on whether people should go to university and whether this is good for society.

Q13: I'm going to show you a painting, imagine that you have been tasked with describing this to someone over the phone so that they can recreate it, but you only have a minute. How would you describe the painting in order to make the recreation as close to the original as possible?

This question is very common and surprisingly difficult. **You can take a number of approaches.** Ensure that you have a concrete idea of the structure you will use to describe the painting. For example, you could begin with your personal feelings about it, then the colours and atmosphere the painting creates, then the exact objects, then their respective position and size. It does not matter which approach you take but this question is designed to test your way of organising and presenting your ideas.

You could also comment on the difficulty of the task and argue that human language limits you from adequately describing smell, taste, sound, and vision. Modern language applicants may have read about Wittgenstein, in which case, they can reference his works on the limitations and functions of language here.

Q14: Which person in the past would you most like to interview, and why?

This is a personal question but try to **avoid generic and mainstream answers**. Keep in mind that you can find out much more about a particular period or era by speaking to everyday citizens or advisors for politicians or other important figures. It is much more important to identify what you want to learn about and then set criteria to narrow down the possible list of persons. This question opens the floor for developing an analytical, quasi-scientific approach to your research.

Q15: What's an interesting thing that's been happening in the news recently?

Whilst this question may be asked at a general interview, it's a good idea to come up with something that is related to your course. Instead of going into technical detail with an interviewer who may be from a completely different discipline, it is better to give a brief overview of the article and then put it into a broader context.

For example, an economics applicant may want to discuss the most recent banking scandal. A physics applicant may want to discuss a recent discovery.

A **good** candidate might say something like "That's a great question, there are a lot of really interesting things which have happened recently. For me, I think the most interesting one is the confirmation of increased magnetic movement in muons at the Fermi National Accelerator in America.

This is mainly interesting for two reasons, I think that it is always interesting when you have examples of the standard model perhaps not working as it should. It's seemed like there have been problems with the way we understand everything working for some time now, but actually being able to perhaps find a new force, and write new laws of physics is incredibly exciting! The other reason this in particular is interesting is because it shows some of the strengths and weaknesses of the scientific process. Even though this magnetic movement has been detected in multiple experiments for over twenty years, it is still not something which we can consider confirmed, because this movement has not been confirmed to the five-sigma level of certainty needed to announce an actual discovery. This rigour helps ensure that we don't have incidents like the Pons and Felischmann Cold Fusion scandal, but does also mean that we will have waited more than two decades to start re-writing the textbooks at the point that this can be confirmed, assuming of course that it ever is. Events like this one really show how thorough and reliable scientific work can be, but also that in areas like theoretical physics things can be very slow to change."

The answer should not be a complete analysis of the issue but an intuitive and logical description of an event, with a good explanation of why it is interesting to you, personally. They really want to see here your enthusiasm for the topic of the article in question (and hopefully the topic of your chosen course) as well as your ability to reflect in a mature way on its most general themes.

Q16: Can people be entirely apolitical? Are you political?

In general, you should avoid expressing any very extreme views at all during interviews. The answer, "I do not" is not the most favourable either. This question invites you to **demonstrate academic thinking in a topic which could be part of everyday conversations**. You are not expected to present a full analysis of party politics and different ideologies. It doesn't matter if you actually have strong political views; the main point is to talk about your perception of what political ideas are present and how one differs from the other.

With such a broad question – you have the power to choose the topic- be it wealth inequality, nuclear weapons, corruption, human rights, or budget deficit etc. Firstly, you should **explain why that particular topic or political theme is important**. For example, the protection of fundamental human rights is crucial in today's society because this introduces a social sensitivity to our democratic system where theoretically 51% of the population could impose its will on the other 49%. On the other hand, it should be noted that Western liberal values may contradict with social, historical and cultural aspects of society in certain developing countries, and a different political discourse is needed in different countries about the same questions. Secondly, you should discuss whether that topic is well-represented in the political discourse of our society and what should be done to trigger a more democratic debate.

Q17: One of the unique features of Oxbridge education is the supervision system, one-on-one tutorials every week. This means a heavy workload, one essay every week with strict deadlines. Do you think you can handle this?

By this point, you should hopefully have a sound understanding of the supervision/tutorial systems. You should also be aware of the possibility of spending long hours in the library and meeting tight deadlines so this question should not be surprising at all. It gives you an opportunity to **prove that you would fit into this educational system very well**. Firstly, you should make it clear that you understand the system and the requirements. On average, there is one essay or problem sheet every week for each paper that you are reading which requires going through the reading list/lecture notes and engaging with wider readings around certain topics or problems. Secondly, you should give some examples from your past when you had to work long hours or had strict deadlines etc. You should also tell the interviewer how you felt in these situations, what you enjoyed the most and what you learned from them. Finally, you may wish to stress that you would not only be able to cope with the system but also enjoy it a great deal.

Q18: If you had to live in the world of a book you have read, which book would it be, and whose role would you take?

This question is an ice-breaker- the interviewer is curious to find out what type of novels you read and how thoroughly you are reading them. You want to show that you are capable of thinking on your feet, talk them through why you've chosen their particular world, does it have advantages which outweigh its pitfalls. For example, if you say you like Robin Hood, it is a world in which you could carry out noble deeds in an idyllic setting, but you also have to deal with poverty, homelessness, and a brutal regime. If you would like to live here, then tell them why. As for the character, centre in on who you want, for instance Robin himself, explain his situation briefly as becoming an outlaw, resisting the authorities, and aiding the poor and his fellow men. Would you like to take his role because you would like to do the things he did, or do you feel that you could 'be' him differently, or even better? Would you be able to learn or grow from entering your chosen world, and being a certain character - think of what course you are applying to, and see if there are particular skills which you think this experience could teach you, empathy, if you're applying for medicine, or social responsibility, if you're applying for economics & management, as examples.

The main point is to be able to **give a very brief summary of the character and the world in which they live**, (especially if you choose a less well-known work), and have a good and interesting justification for choosing them.

Q19: Do you think that we should give applicants access to a computer during their interviews?

This is a classic open question for an insightful debate. The most important thing to realise here is that **Oxbridge education is about teaching you how to think** in clear, structured and coherent ways as opposed to collecting lots of facts from the internet.

Internet access would provide each candidate with the same available information and therefore the art of using information to make sound arguments would be the sole decisive factor. On the other hand, the information overload can be rather confusing. In general, a brain dump is not helpful at the interview as it does not demonstrate in-depth understanding and analysis of any problems. At the end of the day, it comes down to the individual candidate, i.e. what would you look up on the Internet during the interview? Would you want to rely on unverified knowledge? How reliable is that information on the internet? How could you verify this information?

Q20: What was your proudest moment?

This is another chance to highlight your suitability for the course, so try to make it as subject-relevant as possible. "I felt proud to be awarded first place in a poetry competition with a sonnet I wrote about…" (if you're applying for English). "I recently won the Senior Challenge for the UK Mathematics Trust.", "Achieving a 100% mark in my AS-level History and English exams – an achievement I hope to emulate at A2".

Of course, it's not easy to pick one achievement and this is not a question you might have expected. You could also argue that you can't really compare your achievements from different fields e.g. your 100% Physics AS-level and football team captaincy. This will allow you to bypass the question's number limit and mention more than one achievement so that you have more opportunities to impress the interviewer.

Q21: Would you ever use a coin-flip to make a choice, if so, when?

This question can be quite tricky and aims at revealing how you make decisions in your life, your understanding of abstract concepts, rationality and probabilities. You should begin with answering the question from your perspective, you can be honest about it but give a justification even if you never want to make decisions based on luck. Try to **give a few examples when tossing a coin could be a good idea**, or would cause no harm. Then you can take the discussion to a more abstract level and argue that once all yes/no decisions are made by tossing a coin in the long run, the expected value should be fifty-fifty so you might not be worse-off at all and you could avoid the stress of making decisions (although this is very simplistic).

You could also reference the stock markets where high returns may be purely luck-dependent. On the other hand, **rational decision-making is part of human nature** and analysing costs and benefits would result in better decisions in the long-run than tossing a coin. In addition, this would incentivise people to conduct research, collect information, develop and test theories, etc. As you see, the question could be interpreted to focus on the merits of rigorous scientific methodology.

Q22: If you had omnipotence for a moment, but had to use it to change only one thing, what would it be?

This question tests your sound reasoning and clear presentation of your answer and the justification for it. There is no right or wrong "one thing" to choose. It is equally valid to choose wealth inequality or the colour of a double-decker bus if you argue it well! It should be noted that if you've applied for social sciences, it is a better strategy to choose a related topic to show your sensitivity to social issues.

Firstly, you should choose something you would like to change while demonstrating clear thinking, relevant arguments. Secondly, you are expected to discuss how, and to what extent, you would and could change it. Again, a better candidate would realise that **this is not necessarily a binomial problem** – either change it or not – but there may be a spectrum between these two extremes. Once you've identified the thing you'd like to change, talk them through why. A good way to make sure you always do this is by thinking aloud, and walking the interviewer through the way you would reach this conclusion yourself.

Q23: Oxford, as you know, has access to some very advanced technology. In the next room we actually have the latest model of time machine, if we gave you the opportunity to use it later, when would you go?

This is a question where you can really use your imagination (or draw on History GCSE or A-level). **You can say absolutely any time period** in the past or the future but you must have a good reason for it which you communicate to the interviewer. This doesn't necessarily need to be linked to your subject.

For example, *"I would love to see a time when my parents were little children and see where and how they grew up. I'd ideally like to stay for some time to gather as much information as possible. This would be really valuable to me as I'd get to see them when they were people without children, just as they themselves were developing, and could give me opportunities to better understand them. I think understanding one's parents is often a good way to help you understand yourself. The pursuit of self-understanding never stops, but this opportunity would give me a unique chance to improve that."*

Choosing something personal or creative will make you stand out and you are more likely to get interesting questions from the interviewer if you are able to involve them in an intriguing conversation. It is also fine if you choose a standard period like the Roman Empire or a time which has not yet come to pass, say the year 4000, if you have a good reason.

Q24: Should interviews be used for selection?

This question may appear slightly inflammatory on the surface, considering that you are answering it in an interview, to an interviewer who likely believes in the merit of interviewing for selection. However, remember that the interviewer is interested in your opinion, and will not take offence providing you respond in a measured way, providing examples/evidence. Another important thing to remember for any question that addresses interviews and/or selection, is that what you are currently sat in is not the only form of interview, and what you are being selected for is not the only form of selection. As a result, you could wildly disagree with interviews for selection in most situations, but agree with them in the situation you are currently sat in, or vice versa.

"One up-side to using interviews for selection, is that it forces the interviewee to think on their feet (providing the questions aren't known to them in advance), which can demonstrate their real-world knowledge of a subject and is likely to bring out more honest answers about themselves. One down-side is that an interview is quite a short and high-pressure situation, as a result, an interviewee could easily make a number of mistakes or say something inappropriate and tarnish the interviewer's opinion of them. By extension, interviews rely somewhat on the opinion of the interviewer, therefore, are prone to bias."

This would be a good answer, as it addresses one for and one against aspect, justifying each point with an explanation. However, a great answer would be one that takes this further, and considers interviews' appropriateness for different types of selection.

"In some situations, the ability for an interviewee to make a mess of the interview due to the short time they are with the interviewer, and the pressure they are under, is a bad thing. This is in the same way that an entire year's work boiling down to one exam is often criticised as a way of measuring someone's academic ability. However, if the interview is for something that requires working in that situation, such as a politician who will be subjected to questions and interviews throughout their job, then an interview is a great way to measure their suitability."

By considering the appropriateness of an interview in different scenarios, you are not only demonstrating your breadth of consideration, but also your ability to remove yourself from your own head and think outside of your current situation. This question could, however, specify a type of interview and/or a particular thing being selected for. In this case, make sure you stick to that specific concept. You may address an alternative concept for comparison, but always bring the conclusion back to the question's specific elements.

Q25: Would you ever choose to go to a party rather than write an essay for university?

At first glance, this might feel like a trick question. As an interviewer, they are likely a practicing academic at the university and could well be a subject tutor you could end up having! However, it's important to remember two things. Firstly, tutors are human too and like to have fun occasionally. Secondly, all universities have 'parties' that are sanctioned by the university or an individual faculty, therefore, it's perfectly fine to want to go to parties! There are a couple of distinctions to make when constructing an answer for a question like this, and they hinge on the importance of each element.

In isolation, you might consider it impossible to argue that a party is in any way important. However, there are lots of ways in which it could be. This could a big, once in a lifetime faculty ball, it could be a party for a close friend's birthday, it could have valuable networking opportunities, or it could simply be a party you really could do with as you're feeling a bit down at that moment. The other aspect of this question is, of course, the essay. When picking something over something else, you should be considering the importance of each thing in isolation to the current situation, rather than just the concepts in general. For example, if the essay is due tomorrow and the party is a small get-together down the hall which is going to result in you not sleeping properly and not being able to finish the essay in time, then it would be quite difficult (although not impossible in the 'right' circumstances) to argue that you would pick the party over the essay.

Under some circumstances, the party might be a well-deserved break from your work, and not directly impact your ability to submit the essay by the deadline. For example, if an essay is due at the end of the following day and the party is that night, it might initially seem sensible to finish the essay first and relax after. However, you won't be able to go to the party tomorrow afternoon once you've finished the essay, as it won't be going on then. So, in that case, it would make sense to go to the party and then finish the essay the following afternoon before the deadline (providing you have enough time to do so). This sort of decision-making is more likely to go approved by an interviewer if the party has some kind of important element (e.g., a big, one-off organised event or a birthday party), but even if not, it is important to be able to back your decisions. As long as you are completing the work to a high standard and on time, it's also important that you enjoy yourself!

Q26: Who do you think has the most power: Biden, Merkel or Adele?

Answering a question like this first rests on your knowledge of each person. You don't need to know a great deal about them, but it is important you know what their role is. If you don't know that, make sure you ask the interviewer! Once you have established who each person is, you need to address any words in the question that have multiple interpretations. In this case, that word is 'power'. In order to answer the question, you need to decide how to measure power. As with all of these types of questions, you are welcome to pick one definition and go with it, or address the fact that there are multiple definitions and briefly approach each one individually. You can always make a comparison/conclusion at the end of the latter to potentially pick the 'best' definition for that particular situation.

When defining power, there are two key starting points. The first is how many people are aware of what each person says or does. This is probably the easiest to answer.

"If you consider power to be the potential of each person's words or actions to affect others, then the most influential would probably be Adele. Her music and name are known worldwide so, while she is probably not known by as many people in the US as Biden is, her reach is more global and likely through to a younger audience. More people will have heard her, and responded in any number of different ways, even turning off the radio is affecting others. However, as Biden progresses through his presidency and makes more headlines, that could easily change!"

Due to the simplicity of this definition, in this case, it is probably best to address at least one other definition of influence. One alternative definition is how much those who hear what that person says or sees what they do, will change their thoughts or long-term actions based on it.

"If defining power as how much people will change their actions or thoughts based on the actions and words of that person, then the most influential person is probably Biden. As the Amercian president, the majority of the US population will be brought into his words and actions, even if it is to vehemently disagree with them!"

You could go on to explore whether power can be just as valid when someone disagrees with the words or actions of an influential individual, or how many more people would someone need to affect a little bit to make them more powerful than someone who influences a smaller number of people a lot. The important thing is that you explore your thought processes aloud, and see them through to a conclusion each time. The conclusion doesn't need to be right, as with a concept like this it is hard to be 'right', it just needs to be some kind of decision (even if that decision is there is a tie!).

Q27: What would you say was "your colour"?

With a question as basic and seemingly abstract as this, there are two ways you can approach it. The first is to delve into the question in-depth and explore each concept and its origin. The alternative is to answer the question succinctly and give a clear reason for your conclusion. Below is an example of the latter.

"I believe that red is a colour that represents me best as it is my favourite colour. I think it came about as my favourite colour because my parents' car when I was a child was red, as was the front door on the first house I remember living in, so I always associated red with my family and home".

That would be enough detail to give a valid answer. You have given the basis of the reason (that it is your favourite colour), and then discussed the origin of that reasoning. Alternatively, you can choose to explore the question in much more detail. The first concept to approach when doing this, is the idea of representation. Is this self-representation, how others would represent you, or perhaps how you relate to what the colour typically represents in society. Below is an example of a succinct approach to all three of those concepts, something you could state after outlining the three concepts aloud.

"For myself, the colour green represents me best because it is my favourite colour, I own lots of green clothes and decorations in my room and would love to have a green house! If other people had to choose, I'd say they would pick blue because I spent a lot of time in rivers in my parents' canoe, and enjoy spending time in the sea on holiday. If I had to be represented by a societal norm, I would day that red best represents me because I have a fiery temper."

While, in the real interview you would probably approach each of these in a bit more details, this gives a basic outline of how you would separate the three concepts. You don't have to address every concept in your answer but, as usual, it is always good to outline all the concepts in the beginning to demonstrate to the interviewer that you are thinking comprehensively. Remember, when you are addressing multiple concepts in an answer, it is all too easy to drift away from the origin of your thoughts. Bring it back each time by answering the actual question at the end of each of your thought processes, in the context that thought process has been discussed in.

Q28: What shape is man? What shape is time?

On the surface, this question seems impossible to answer because it is simply too abstract. There is no shape that fits the shape of a person, and time isn't a physical concept. However, this is a test of how you address something seemingly impossible to answer. There is no wrong way to answer this question, providing you actually answer it! The important thing to remember is to get started with answering it quickly, the longer you spend pondering the wider concept, the more difficult it will be to get started!

Addressing each question individually is important and something you need to conclude on so, as a result, it is easy for you to separate two concept discussions by addressing one per question. When considering the first question, you can start by providing the obvious answer, and follow-on by delving into the concept more deeply.

"There is no named shape that is the shape of a person, so you would refer to 'man' simply as being 'man-shaped'. We refer to things in this way all the time, so not having a named shape to represent something shouldn't limit you. One important differentiator is that 'man' is not an exact shape, as every person is different. Therefore, if your definition of shape must be precise such as a square having four equal length sides with four ninety-degree corners, then that would not be possible to apply to 'man'. However, a shape like an oval doesn't have explicit parameters, so is closer to the idea of a shape which could define 'man'."

There are clear caveats to this answer, such as an oval having the strict rule of no straight edges and being entirely symmetrical, but the consideration of two different types of existing shape definitions is a great way to start the discussion. When moving that discussion on to consider time, it becomes even more abstract. You could open the discussion with the fact that time is not considered a physical concept, thus it would be inappropriate to allocate it a shape. However, you then open the discussion around space-time, where time can be considered represented physically. An interviewer may not choose to entertain such a discussion, as it is not exactly psychology related, but making sweeping and abrupt statements like that are best avoided anyway. A better way to open the discussion might be to explain that time is often considered a circle (history repeating itself, the circle of life etc.). While it would be inappropriate to state that time is a specific shape, acknowledging these ideas demonstrates your ability to think conceptually and compare it to real societal discussion.

Q29: Do things have to have specific names?

When answering why, the first thing to consider is 'what's in it for the user'. In this case, what is gained by naming things.

"One reason why things have names is to avoid having to describe them every time we refer to them. Once you have learned what the name refers to, conversations can be had much more quickly, and more easily across different languages. Rather than having to learn all the terms that describe a thing, you would only need to learn the name of that thing in order to tell a person about it in a different language."

You can centre the entire discussion around this idea of what we gain from something, but it is important to broaden your horizons a little if you want to make the discussion as interesting and engaging as possible. You may consider a few gains we make by naming things, but the next step is to consider the origin of naming things and the reason for the concept. The first reason is that we gain something from doing it, so it justifies the effort of coming up with and learning the names, However, another example which would explain the origin of naming something is that we want to take ownership of it. By giving something a name, it can be recognised by that name and associated with one person as its 'owner'. This could be considered the origin of naming, whereby everyone would have a different name for the few things they considered to be there. Gradually, through communication, perhaps we established it would be easier to have a unified naming process, such that there were fewer names to remember. This could have led to the origin of possessive pronouns, to go with these unified names.

None of this is necessarily true, and would be almost impossible to prove either way due to how long-ago naming things came about as a concept. Discussions of this type do, however, demonstrate your ability to consider both the value and the origin of a concept or action and link them together. The importance of a question like this, is to evoke a discussion of the abstract that you can tie together into a coherent conclusion. As such, it is vital that regardless of the content of your discussion, you conclude with an actual answer. This is welcome to be a brief touch of each of the discussion points you have made, as it is often impossible to make an explicit decision on which is 'right', but it needs to be clear and concise.

"I believe things have names because it was a way of identifying them as our own, which developed into a way of communicating what they were between people who didn't know of each other's possessions. It stuck as a concept, because it enabled shorter discussions through not having to fully describe a thing each time it was mentioned."

Q30: Do you read any international publications, do you think there is a value to doing so?

This question requires honesty above all else. This doesn't mean you couldn't implicitly overstate quite to the extent that you read a particular publication, but you absolutely should not discuss something you haven't actually read. Many of the interviewers you will speak to will ask this question because they are very well read, thus could easily pull you up on a particular publication. As a result, you need to have actually read an international newspaper or publication to answer this question. It would be best if you have read at least one of each, but if you have only read one, open with that.

What the interviewer will be looking for is your critique of the publication. It would be a bonus if it is psychology-related, but don't think it to be necessary. The important thing is that you recognise and address the context under which the publication is written, and how that might influence what they write about and how they write about it. When critiquing an academic paper in an essay, these are the sorts of things a tutor will be looking to see, and it is what the interviewer wants to assess your ability on at this stage. This isn't to say that you should construct your entire discussion of the publication around this critiquing, but it is definitely something you should include.

"I read [American Newspaper] online quite regularly, and tend to focus on the 'social issues' section of the paper. It is interesting to read about American social issues because some of them are so similar to our own, whereas others are so distinctly different. One article I read in the most recent version [don't be this specific if you're not sure it was] *highlighted the ease with which someone could buy a gun as a non-American citizen, meaning that someone who's history is unknown to American authorities could enter the country and buy a weapon with bad intentions. I wonder whether gun culture contributes to xenophobia and racism, as the risk that someone coming into the country with bad intentions poses, is potentially much higher than if the same thing happened where guns weren't accessible to the public."*

While this is a very simplistic discussion of a point and you would want to delve into some more detail and evidence in the real interview, it demonstrates how you can bring a psychology them to a seemingly unrelate article. The next stage in your discussion would be to critique the paper itself. With gun culture being alien to a UK resident (if indeed you are one), you could consider your views on the topic to be biased. You could also make a suggestion to rectify that, by discussing the article with an American person or someone who is in favour of guns being legally accessible to the public. This last bit is important as it is key to consider how you can broaden your views in a practical way. If the context is right, you can link it to how you might do this during your time at university.

Q31: Can you hear silence?

There are two elements that can be considered in almost any question which touches on biology in a psychology interview. The first is the biological element, and the second is the concept that we experience/express as a result or in anticipation of that biological effect. In this case, there is the biology of hearing something, and the interpretation of that into neural signals. In this case, how you explain the biology is very much dependent on your biology knowledge. Unless it is something you have mentioned in your personal statement or in the interview, the interviewer won't expect you to have comprehensive knowledge of the biology behind hearing. However, they will expect you to have a general understanding that sound travels in waves, and those waves are interpreted into neural signals (which we 'hear') by bones in your ear.

When considering this from a biological perspective, then you can be pretty conclusive in your statement that we cannot hear silence. If there are no sound waves, then we do not 'hear' anything from our environment. However, this doesn't mean that we don't interpret the silence as something other than nothingness, from the neural signals we receive. Without making any sweeping statements about the complicated biology around neural signalling, it would make sense to assume that neurons aren't ever 'silent'. Things in biology are rarely as cut and dry as being 'off' or 'on', so you could use that train of thought in the following discussion.

"I imagine that neurons are never at a point when there is no transmission of chemical between them. It is more likely to imagine they have a 'resting rate' of transmission, which is then greatly increase when 'active'. As a result, even when there is no noise, you might assume there are still some signals being sent between neurons related to hearing. In order to create a silent environment, humans have gone to great lengths to create sound-deadening material. Therefore, one could assume that silence is not something you would come across in a natural setting. If the human hearing system has not evolved to consider true silence, when faced with it, its reaction will likely be to 'hear' the 'resting rate' of signals that would normally never be reached due to ambient noise. With that in mind, while you cannot actually hear silence because there are no sound waves to hear, the experience of true silence is likely to manifest as some kind of ambient sound."

Making one point per statement in a discussion like this enables you to create an argument that is easy to follow. This is beneficial for three reasons. Firstly, the interviewer can take note of every point you have made. Secondly, the interviewer can see you are proficient at organising your thoughts. Thirdly, the interviewer can be invited to target a new discussion (even if that is to disagree with you) at any one of your points. The more discussion the better!

Q32: You mentioned having good thinking skills in your personal statement, can you tell me how many golf balls can you fit in a Boeing 787 Dreamliner?

This question is testing a few things, all related to your thinking process, despite its seemingly pointless nature. The first thing it is testing is the comprehensiveness and commitment of your subject consideration. What the interviewer will be looking for is you to exhaust all aspects of the question, in order to work towards the answer. Part of this is considering the physical nature of the objects in mind. The two elements in this question are the plane, and the golf balls. To consider the physical size of the plane, it might be best to get some clarification from the interviewer if you don't know the size of the plane. The number will be very different between a double-decker transatlantic plane compared to a private jet! If you know the size, make sure you state it out loud, it doesn't really matter whether you are right or not, just that the interviewer knows what you are working from. When discussing the golf ball, make sure you also give the rough size you are working from.

The next step has two options. The first is to take a mathematical approach, based around volume. The other is to consider all the places you could put a golf ball on a plane (overhead storage, under seats, in cockpit etc.). Depending on your maths confidence, the choice would be yours. Don't worry if the maths you do isn't exactly right, just make sure you talk through each step out loud and ensure that the number you come out with at the end seems believable. If working through the different places a ball could go, try to attribute a number to each one (e.g., 300 golf balls in each overhead storage area, 300 passengers so 100 areas, 30000 total golf balls in overhead storage), and make sure you write it down! It's far too easy to get caught up in the line of sums, without being able to add them together to an answer at the end!

Once you reach a point of concluding, ensure that your answer appears believable and answer the question! Don't let yourself tail off at the end of your last consideration and not actual provide a number. It doesn't matter (within reason) what that number is, as long as the methods you used to get to it made sense.

Q33: How would you work out the number of flights passing over London at this moment?

This question is testing just one thing, that being the degree to which you can work through a large series of thoughts, considering all possible options. While it is vital that you give a numerical answer, the value of that answer (within reason) doesn't really matter, what matters is how you got to the answer. When beginning this question, it might be helpful for you to outline some parameters. If you know how many airports London has (6), then you can start from there. There will definitely be more than 6 planes over London as they will be coming and going from each airport. So, from your starting point you can work out a realistic maximum.

If you know anything about airport scheduling then absolutely discuss it, any colourful insights into your life will be memorable for an interviewer. However, most people won't have that kind of insight so will be starting from scratch. It would be safe to assume that there is a gap of at least two minutes between planes landing, in order that they can taxi off of the runway. At the speed planes travel, they could probably traverse London in 15 minutes or so. Considering of the 6 airports, there are maybe 10 runways, assuming planes are always nose to tail coming in and out, you could sum 7 planes per 'queue' times the 10 runways, making a total of 70 planes.

It doesn't matter if this is entirely wrong, it may be hugely more than this or hugely fewer. The important thing is the steps taken to get to that value. If you want to extend your discussion, you can go on to review the number you have reached. If you look up at the sky at any given time, you can only see a couple of planes at most, and your view extends quite a few miles in every direction. As such, you might choose to assess that 70 seems like too many, and perhaps halve your answer. If you add in the explanation that maybe there is a 4-minute gap between landings, rather than the originally assumed 2, the numbers would add up. Being comprehensive and explanatory in your thought processes is vital and will be most well received by an interviewer.

Q34: How many deliveries are made in the UK every day?

As with any numerical question, the value is your method, not the answer. However, you must give an answer to 'complete' the process. To reach any kind of answer to the scale that this will be will take some considerable calculations. If you have any prior insight (such as knowing how many they delivered last year, or how many your local post office receives), then outline and apply it aloud. Each bit of information you can bring to inform your calculation will not only likely make it more accurate, but also impress the interviewer that you have such niche knowledge and have thought to apply it.

When starting your calculations, it can be helpful to set parameters. You can assume that not every person in the UK receives something every day, so the number is likely going to be less than the total UK population (if you know it accurately, great, if not it can be generally helpful to know it's around 70 million people). Your next point of consideration is that commercial mail exists as well. While much of mail is sent via email now, businesses still account for a lot of the mail sent each day. As such, you may choose to reconsider your original 70-million limit, to account for commercial mail.

None of the assumptions and considerations you make matter in their accuracy to reality, only in their abundance and degree of thought. Within reason, in a question like this, the more times you reconsider a particular point, the greater depth of understanding it demonstrates to the interviewer. When you have made all the considerations you think are reasonable (it can be helpful to write them down to keep track), make sure you conclude with an actual value. Once you have a value, it can often be insightful to reflect upon that relative to a reasonable assumption you might pick out of the air. If this calculated value and the 'random' value are distinctly different, perhaps spend a moment discussing why that might be, relative to the calculations and considerations you have just undertaken.

Q35: Have you been to this college before?

This question is unusual, in that it is not testing anything in particular. It is far more of an exploratory question which seeks to bring out your experience of university and the college, as well as your expectations for it going forward. When answering any question based on your experiences, it is important to be honest. You can embellish the truth in part if you wish, but always ensure that the core of what you're saying is true. The interviewer will probably expect you to have visited Oxford at least once before the interview (unless you are an international student), but it is not a problem if you have not.

If you have not ever visited the college before, the interviewer will want to know what attracted you to it, and that will likely be the next question. As a result, your considerations should immediately be looking towards why you were interested in the college, as soon as this initial question is asked. The best way to approach that, is to describe in what context you have seen the college (e.g., through the university website) and what it was that you liked about what you saw/read.

If you have visited the college before, the first thing to outline is under what context. If it was a family trip to Oxford and you looked around as a tourist, it is fine to focus on the 'tourist things' that you liked about the college e.g., the architecture. If you visited quite recently (during the time you might be expected to have been thinking about university) or as a school trip, where the focus was a little more on the academic side, then make sure you address some of the 'non-tourist- aspects too. It is fine to talk about the grounds and the architecture, but having done some reading around the library, subject foci and alumni/faculty members will go a long way.

 This is one of the few questions where it wouldn't really be fitting to conclude by answering the question. Answering the question should be the very first thing you do, everything that follows is simply an extension of that. One key thing to make sure is that you don't end up talking too far into the subject. It may be that the interviewer was simply asking this as a yes/no question, precursory to a more in-depth question. With that in mind, try to read the interviewer's body language to see if they were expecting you to take the reins on the discussion!

Q36: Do you think that Oxford/Cambridge will suit you?

This question is testing two main things. The first is your understanding of (and, by extension, your reading up on) the university, and your self-awareness. You want to ensure that the overriding message of this answer is 'yes', as that is the whole reason you are applying. However, don't be afraid to touch on some elements that may not be 100% positive. For example, if you feel like you don't have much in common with the stereotypical student of the university, you can say that! However, what is important is to express your realisation that the stereotype isn't the reality.

If you want to go down this route of discussion, the safest is way to is to describe your experiences once you have arrived. By the time you have gone into your first interview, you will have had quite extensive contact with some other prospective students. More than likely, you will have found some people with things in common with yourself, take that on board I your discussion. The more recent the experience and the more truth behind it, the better! If this process of meeting your fellow interviewees has squashed some doubt about whether you would fit in, that's a fantastic result and you should definitely share it!

The next part is to make sure that you have read up on the university, and to make that clear! If the university is very research heavy, match that up to your own academic interests! The same goes for if they have a particular department that is of interest to you. Don't be afraid to add a little more personality to the discussion, perhaps the location is convenient for you in some way, but make sure your answer hinges on the more impactful content.

"After my undergraduate degree, I would really enjoy pursuing a PhD in psychology. I'm not sure exactly what I would want to specialise in yet, but the opportunity to be surrounded by practicing academics to discuss that with is invaluable. In addition, I'll be able to stay on my undergraduate campus for my postgraduate studies, and have access to some incredible research facilities and equipment. In addition, the university is only 45 minutes' drive from my home town, so I'll be able to visit there easily for birthdays and other special occasions!"

Remember, this question is about why the university is the right fit for you. You could easily be asked why you are the right fit for the university, and you would have to phrase your answer slightly differently. To explain why the university is the right fit for you, you should be assessing why the features of the university fit into your life and personality. If you're answering why you're the right fit for the university, then that answer is the other way round!

Q37: What do you think you'll be doing in a decade? How about in two decades?

No interviewer will expect you to have an actual plan for the next 10 or 20 years of your life. Instead, what they're looking for is an understanding of how you gaining your degree might set out a path for you in life. This is far more about understanding your options than it is deciding which one you are going to pursue. It is important to distinguish the sections of your answer between the 10 and 20-year mark. Remember if you wanted to do a PhD, you wouldn't likely finish that until around 8 years from the point that you're in this interview. As such, if that was your plan, you wouldn't be far into post-doctoral research/your first 'proper' job in the first 10 years. It is important to articulate details like this, even if you haven't definitely decided you want to do a PhD. Any understanding of your options in this way demonstrates to the interviewer that you have considered these things.

If you are more concerned with the industry you want to go into than any postgraduate studies, then discuss how you might want to pursue success there. At the 10-year point, if you have spent 6 years of that in an industry, what would you like to have achieved. You have the classic milestones such as being a team leader, running your own project, owning your own home, or any other 'standard' aspirations. However, you should try and add in some things which are unique to you and your preferred industry. If you wanted to go into marketing, something that is quite common for psychology graduates, then it would be great to aspire to have one of your projects on national television, or up in the store of a 'household name' business.

It is, however, important to remember that the interviewer is likely to be an academic, and is likely to (be it potentially implicitly/subconsciously) want you to aspire to do the same thing. As a result, you should consider how you 'tune' your answer to appease those who are listening to it. I would never expect a tutor to reject an applicant on the basis that they didn't want to pursue studies beyond undergraduate, however, it is easier to engage with someone on a topic they are interested in. The more engaged you are with the interviewer, the more likely they will remember and the better a conversation they will have with their peers after you are gone. This isn't a hard and fast rule, but it is human nature to frame memorable things in a positive light (unless of course it was objectively bad!). in sum, you want to approach this question with honesty, but make sure that you consider your audience!

Q38: What is your favourite activity outside of school?

This is a question which 'assesses' your personality outside of academia. It's great if you have genuine hobbies which are subject-related, but most people don't and no interviewer will expect you to. What they are looking for is ways in which you unwind, what environments you choose to put yourself in (rather than those which are thrust upon you!), and how competitive you are. If every hobby of yours involves playing a competitive, spectator sport to a high level, then the interviewer can deduce that you are outgoing, competitive and have an interest in exhibiting your skills. This is very different (although by no means better/worse) than someone who's hobbies are all quiet activities to pass the time that you engage with alone.

As you discuss your interests, remember that the interviewer will likely be comparing their stereotypical view of someone who has these interests, alongside their experience of you in this setting. If you are describing yourself as confident and outgoing through the activities you like to do, but are aware that you have been shy in this setting, it could be a good thing to highlight that! Having a high level of self-awareness is a great sign of emotional intelligence and will only be another point in your favour!

When talking about your interests, it is always beneficial to highlight any achievements you might have made in them. This doesn't mean you should tune the entire conversation into a list of your achievements (as that wasn't the question!), but it can be useful to highlight where you have committed yourself and gained success. In addition, spend some time on the less usual hobbies. This is the perfect opportunity to inject some real personality into the interview and, you never know, the interviewer might even share an unusual hobby of yours which you can engage on!

Lastly, it can be a good idea to describe how you are going to continue pursuing those hobbies through university. The interviewers don't want someone who is going to drop everything and become a sheep when they arrive on campus, they want someone who is going to bring something new to the table! As a result, whether it's simply a hobby you'll keep up in your own time, or a club that you'd want to set up in your college, make sure you outline how you'll go about keeping these things up! Make sure these are realistic and measured against the amount of commitment you will need to bring to your academic studies, but by all means dream big!

Q39: How will your fellow college residents see you?

There are a few ways in which you can contribute to college life as a student. One, which could be easily overlooked when considering college life specifically, is simply being a friendly and approachable person. When talking in the context of college life, it's easy to forget the things that make you a contributor to a pleasant society in general. When it comes to college-specific things, it's good to open with some more general points, with some demonstration that you have read up on college-specific things as well.

What this means is first considering what makes a good contributor in any small community. You could contribute by applying your skills in a particular sport (or otherwise) to the college team, you could apply your academic ability and commitment to success to enhance the college's academic rankings. You could even include something like experience in party-planning or finances to contribute to the college ball (should there be one). The next step is to introduce some college-specific things, to demonstrate that you've done some reading around the college, and to highlight your specific suitability.

An easy (although predictable) one would be if the college has any particularly successfully (or perhaps even unsuccessful, although that would be more difficult to find out!) sports teams. You could highlight this if you have an interest/skill in any one of those, and highlight that you would be keen to join in. Some of the less predictable things would be societies outside of sport, or whether your college has a chapel and you'd like to be involved in that. There is a wealth of different things which a college could be interested in having someone contribute to, it's just a case of matching one up from your research to something you're interested in. The important thing to remember is that it doesn't have to be something you have dine already, it could be trying something totally new!

Lastly, you want to make sure you can contribute to the college after you leave. Something that many people wouldn't consider is going on to be a respectable and successful person in your industry, adding to the college's notable alumni. As with any question that requires you to speak well of the college/university, it is a fine balance between selling yourself as an admirer of the college, and seeming over the top or fake. Strike the balance well by practicing talking around these kinds of subjects, you'll soon develop a way that works for you.

Q40: Why do you think we structure the course in the way that we do?

This question doesn't try to hide what it's assessing at all. One of the big indicators of someone who is committed to the application process (and, by extension, the university) is how much preparation they have done for the interviews. The first thing you should have looked at when deciding which course to choose, is what the actual course content in. There are two sides to a course decision, the first is how it will help you get to the next stage if your education/career (if you have planned that far ahead!), and the other is whether it will interest you while you study. The latter can only be answered by exploring and reading around the course content.

When talking about the course structure, it is best to keep the objective details to a reasonable level. You don't want to sound like you're simply reciting a list of modules, nor do you want to risk getting muddled and saying something that is objectively wrong. You are much better off making a point which you have come to the opinion of through your reading, and then evidencing it in the discussion thereafter.

"I can see from reading up on the course that it focusses a lot on social psychology in the first two years. This was one of the things that attracted me to it, as I think undertaking a social science independent study in third year would be really interesting. The focus on social psychology seems to come from the disproportionately high number of modules which approach topics in the field, when compared to subjects like perception."

Above is a bit of a clunky answer, but one that demonstrates you've read around the course content and are very happy with what you have read (which is arguably the most important bit!). You could construct an answer in a more coherent manner, by opening with the number of modules on one particular subject, highlighting that it appears to be a particular focus of the course, and then finishing with why that is a good thing for you. However, when opening with the number of modules on a course, it sets up the answer to feel too over-prepared. Your preference between them is, of course, your own and either will make a good structure to answer a question like this.

As aforementioned, the most important bit is to highlight why the course content works for you. Make sure to not have that as the conclusion of your answer, because that isn't the question, but always make sure it is included.

Q41: What would you say was your single greatest weakness?

Answering this question well is very difficult. There are two ways in which you could go wrong. Neither of these ways would necessarily be terrible, but they are best avoided if possible. The first way is to give an answer that is simply a positive attributed in disguise. An example of this would be 'admitting' that you can sometimes be too much of a perfectionist or be too detail oriented. These are things which would certainly be bad traits under certain circumstances, but the combination of the fact that in a lot of cases they are good and that they have been presented as 'sometimes' being an issue, makes them far too weak as answers.

The other way in which you could answer this question in a non-ideal way is to overshare on your weaknesses. The interviewer doesn't want to hear that as soon as there's a test around the corner you have a complete meltdown and only just drag yourself through. If your weakness has something to do with an event you'll face at university, you're best-off underselling it slightly (only if it's really bad of course!). if this is the case, it would also be beneficial to explain what you're doing, and will continue to do, to work on that weakness. Self-awareness of a real weakness is a great sign of the potential for personal growth, but the growth only comes if you actually act to solve the problem!

In an ideal scenario, you will have a genuine weakness that you are working on fixing, that doesn't really have anything to do with university. That way, you can have an honest conversation with the interviewer, without it having any chance of jeopardising their view of you as a competent student. However, this isn't normally possible and you will likely have to talk around a weakness that could affect you as a student.

As a result, you want to focus on what you are doing to rectify this weakness, and the timeline over which you are acting. The latter is very important, no interviewer will expect you to start university as a perfectly formed student, but they would be very keen to see some kind of commitment from you to have worked on that weakness prior to starting your course. It might be that you know you're a slow typist, so you're going to take a touch-typing course over summer. Or it could be that your handwriting is bad quality, so you're going to spend your last few months at school comparing your handwriting every week and looking to see an improvement over time.

There's any number of things you could list as a weakness, just remember that it needs to be honest (and an actual weakness!) but something that is fixable (or at least manageable) in a sensible time-frame.

Q42: You have mentioned a number of personal strengths in your statement, which is your greatest?

Answering this question involves just as much care as answering what your biggest weakness is. It is far too easy to list a generic skill like 'essay-writing' and explaining how it will benefit you in your degree because that is something you will spend a lot of your time doing. The key to answering this question well is finding a balance between bragging and being too modest. If you undersell your strengths, it demonstrates a lack of confidence and perhaps an indication that you might not be as good as you appeared on paper. Oversell your strengths, and it suggests a lack of self-awareness and an arrogance towards your own ability.

To balance this answer properly, you want to find a couple of strengths to 'warm-up' with, that are related to your main strength. Alternatively, you can find one main strength that is backed up with 'auxiliary' strengths. Here is an example of the former, followed by the latter.

"Leading up to my GCSE's, I spent a lot of time doing creative writing in my spare time. I was able to apply those skills and experiences to my English work, as well as my longer answer questions in other subjects. Through all that, I've built up a keen interest and strong ability to write engaging texts on a wide range of topics, making me a good essay-writer. I would say this is my biggest strength in academia."

"My biggest strength in academia is essay-writing. I enjoyed writing through school and wrote lots of stories as a child. By the time I got to my GCSE's my experience and developed proficiency enabled me to excel in English, and at the longer-answer questions in other subjects. I have continued this success into my A-Levels, securing a really good grade in English."

Both of those answers highlight the same strength, but present it in a different way. The latter is for those who are more comfortable 'selling' themselves, the former for those who struggle more with that. One important thig to note is that moth answers highlighted this as being a strength in academia. If you are going to pick that, it is totally fine, but I would open with a statement that highlights it. The interviewers know that you are more than what you can do at school, so will often be looking for non-academic strengths to answer a question like this. If you highlight in the beginning that it is specifically an academic strength, then it prompts them to ask if you have considered a non-academic one too. If you have, feel free to explain that you opened with the one you did because it is your biggest strength, and then explain your other one.

If you want to go ahead and discuss a non-academic strength, of course feel free to do so! It is often easier to add personality in this way, but is sometimes harder to evidence how you have been strong. However, if you use a similar structure, you should be able to present it as a convincing strength.

Q43: How will your experiences from the Duke of Edinburgh scheme benefit you during your time at university?

This is a question that many interviewers will be keen to ask, if you have something like a Duke of Edinburgh mention on your CV/in your personal statement. It may sound a little like they are trying to belittle the achievement by asking it in a sarcastic way, or to try and trip you up. Rest assured that is not the case, they are simply interested to see how you view the skills you have acquired through the program, and how you would apply them to the entirely different environment of studying for a degree.

The key to answering this question well, while it seems obvious, is picking out genuinely applicable skills and experiences. This means valuing relevance over and above the extent of your experience/skill. If you try to shoehorn a skill to fit your university studies, just because it was a large focus of your scheme, your answer will come across ill-fitting. It is important to be prepared for a question like this because it is quite likely to come up, if it is something you have discussed in your personal statement or have on your CV, and it is something quite difficult to come up with off the cuff.

To establish will skill to select, it is best to consider what you have actually done compared to what you will be doing in your degree. If you spent time orienteering and doing crafts, that's not something that fits the bill, however big a part of the scheme it was or how much you enjoyed it. However, if you spent one of the nights up on your own, devising a plan of action and getting everything ready for the following morning, that is something that can be very easily applied to your degree.

"On the last night before our long walk, our team remained very disorganised and we still hadn't got a route fully together, or decided exactly what we needed to pack. I decided, rather than have a frantic rush in the morning, to work into the evening and night to prepare the map route and set up a packing list for each of our team. I had to do this on my own as the rest of my team were getting early nights, so had to rely on my own intuition and conviction behind my decisions. Even though I was tired the next day, I was happy that we were able to set off with a clear route and could have all of our things packed without having to think about whether anything important was missing. I think having to work late, on my own and being able to make those independent decisions has prepared me for the independent projects I will have to take on in my degree."

You could easily have continued the explanation further, regarding the applicability of skills and experience to situations in degree studies, but this demonstrates how you can apply the experience of one isolated event, better than you could trying to apply an irrelevant experience. Remember that the relevance is so much more important than the abundance. It is much easier to oversell how big a deal the event was, than oversell how applicable it is to your degree!

Q44: Why choose Oxford or Cambridge, if you know that other universities are less competitive, and may mark your work much more generously?

There are two ways to approach this question. You can answer successfully discussing one or both. The first point you could make is that you may not actually do better elsewhere. You will likely have spoken in that interview, previous interviews or your personal statement, about how the environment of your chosen university will give you the drive to push forward and excel. At a university where perhaps that drive is not present to the same degree, you may not be pushed in the same way. This is a tricky answer to phrase, as you don't want to come across like you are unable to self-motivate, but if you feel like it applies to you then convincingly portraying that self-awareness will be received well. However, if you don't feel confident discussing that, or it doesn't apply to you, then there is the bulk of the answer to approach.

When answering the main part of this question, you need to consider the value of the university beyond the grade on your degree. If you are confident in yourself that you can achieve a first class result regardless, then that's great. It wouldn't necessarily be the best structure to lead with that, as it would be easy for that to appear arrogant. However, it is a good way to round off your answer, if you are confident talking about that. Approaching the value of the university is all about understanding what it will bring you along the way. If you want to be an academic at that university, then the grade relative to any other university is not really relevant. If you want to learn about your field in the most all-encompassing way possible, then the grade you get is not really relevant to that part of the experience.

However, it is important to acknowledge that as something you have considered. Expressing that awareness will be well-received by an interviewer. The key is to balance it against the personal points you are making. You may wish to make those points after acknowledging your concern around the topic, or you may wish to save it until the end, rounding it off as something that has been weighed up and dismissed based on your conclusion. Most importantly, you should demonstrate that you have the self-confidence to know you can do well in any environment, and not feel the need to establish a different one.

Q45: Cambridge is very intense; do you think your current approach to time management will be sufficient?

There are lots of ways in which you can say you will manage your time. However, the interviewer is going to have heard them all before. The way to make your answer convincing and stand out, is to give evidence of where you have learned these techniques and where you have successfully applied them. It would be a good idea to pick a few techniques for organisation, stress management and timekeeping (although there will. Be some overlap with organisation), and prepare some examples for when these techniques have worked for you in the past. While it would likely make your answer too convoluted if you tried to do this for every technique, it can inject some personality into the answer if you talk about where you learned one of the techniques, particularly if the story is interesting!

"One challenge I am sure that I will face is having to prioritise work. In this sort of situation, it's important to manage explicit deadlines, as well as the importance of each piece of work. During sixth form, I have been a private tutor. Having to manage marking my students' work and completing my own has been very challenging at times. I have mostly chosen to prioritise my students' work, as I have already had discussions with my teachers and they are happy to be lenient with my deadlines, providing they are not exams or coursework!"

By giving a real and honest example of a difficult situation, you'll connect with the tutors a lot better than if you try to make something up on the spot. Once you have explained the situation and experience, as above, it is then important to explicitly apply this to your degree experience.

"From this experience, I am confident talking to tutors and asking them for help with my schedule. In order to stop myself getting too stuck, I would make sure I reach out to a tutor when in need, and ask them to extend my deadline. I would make sure that I am prioritising the work that leads on to future work, so that I don't fall behind on a series of pieces."

By demonstrating your understanding of how you might prioritise something, this gives the interviewer further evidence to suggest what you are saying is something you actually have had to do. In addition, you are showing the confidence to stand up for your decisions, even if that means asking for help.

Q46: What have you read in the last 24 hours?

As with any question that asks you directly about an event, honesty is the best policy. However, it is completely realistic to assume that you may not have read anything on the morning of your interview, or the night before apart from your interview preparation notes. With that in mind, consider this question to be asking more 'what have you read very recently', rather than specifically this morning. That is, unless you have the confidence to be fully honest when, by all means, be exactly that! If you are going to be entirely honest, just ensure that you're not wandering down the road of oversharing. Remember, while the interviewers are friendly and they want to have a pleasant conversation, they are still assessing you! Saying something like "I've actually not read anything in the last 24 hours, I've been a little busy, but just the other day I read some of *The Count of Monte Cristo* in my spare time" is a good way to remain honest while still giving the interviewer something to play off, and giving you something you can explore in depth.

You should make sure you discuss a text you have read recently, and ensure that your discussion is realistic. The interviewer is not going to believe that you have spent your entire morning reading the full works of a particular psychologist, or a novel from cover to cover! The best approach to picking a text is to have read something very recently in preparation for your interviews, and discuss that! If the text is relevant to your interviews, then there's no real reason to spend a lot of time highlighting its relevance. However, if the text is a little more unusual, then by all means explain its relevance to the interviews.

If you choose to discuss a text that has nothing to do with interviews, that's fine too! The interviewer will appreciate the fact that you're reading for pleasure, not just for work! However, the text you discuss should either have an element of psychology, or an element of personality to it, for maximum impact in the interview discussion. The more you can recall about what you read, the better. That's not to say you should go about reciting it verbatim, but it enables you to discuss its content with confidence. If you open with a single point about the text after a brief description of its context, the interviewer may ask you to expand or continue, in which case that gives you the starting point from which to begin your full discussion. If they don't respond in any way to your initial point, try to make you second point psychology related. It may be that they are simply interested to know what you have read recently; in which case they may not pry beyond your initial description. Don't worry either way, all interviewers are different in the way they will want to explore what you have read and how you interpret it.

Q47: What would you say was your greatest personal challenge in life? How did you handle it?

This question is supremely personal, and you should make your answer as such. In an ideal world, you will have had a challenge which comes to mind immediately and you will have no need to prepare any thought on it at all. However, in most people's lives, there are a large number of small challenges, rather than one outstanding one. In this case, the thought you should put into this question is regarding how you overcame one of those challenges. The interviewer is looking to understand a bit more about your background, and build knowledge on how you deal with difficult situations. If you have a challenge that was not quite as big as your biggest ever challenge, but you handled getting over it in a much better way, then that might be your better bet to pick!

As with any of these personal questions, depending on your confidence, you may choose to be 100% honest. It may be that the biggest challenge you have faced was one that you did not overcome well, one that may have beaten you. That is completely fine, as long as you talk about what you learned from that experience. It is no good discussing a difficult situation that wasn't handled well, and then simply going on with your life as if nothing happened! The interviewer will be looking for honesty, self-awareness, self-reflection and the ability to better yourself after a setback. It will be very common for you to come across aa seemingly impassable challenge in your degree, so the interviewer wants to know what experience you have dealing with that kind of situation.

If there is an element of independence to your overcoming of the challenge, highlight that it might be that due to not having the support you might have had in other situations, you didn't handle the challenge as effectively as you might have otherwise. That's fine, but highlight what you learned from the experience and how you would go about approaching it differently next time! It is vital that there is at least an element of self-reflection in your answer. It might be that the challenge happened very recently, and you haven't had enough tie to process it and become better at tackling situations like it. It might be that your biggest challenge was preparing for this interview! If this is the case, then make sure you reflect on that. Don't be afraid to put yourself on the spot to evoke some more honesty out of your answer.

There are three stages to a good answer in this question; situation, specific challenge (and why it was challenging) and what you did/would do next time to overcome it.

Q48: Do you think that the impact of a good teacher can stretch beyond the walls of a school? Who do you think was your best teacher?

Of course, it doesn't matter who your best teacher was, it certainly doesn't need to be the one who is teaching you the subject you're applying for! What matters is how you have assessed them to be your best teacher, and the extent to which you understand how they have influenced you. A poor answer is one that doesn't address any of these elements in any detail, as follows.

"My favourite teacher was my year9 maths teacher. She inspired me to do better in maths and got me from really struggling at the beginning of the year, to being almost top of the class by the end, and really enjoying it!"

A better answer, is one that considers each element of the question in some detail, with a degree of reflection into why you have the thoughts that you do. Below is an answer that does this.

"My favourite teacher was my yr9 maths teacher. She inspired me to do better at maths by simply letting me get on with it, my teachers in years before had always tried so hard to engage me in the lesson when working on the board, and as a shy student I just shrank away and disengaged from the lesson. As soon as I was left to my own devices, I realised I could do it when I wasn't put on the spot! Since then, my confidence grew a lot and by the end of the year I was asking to go through things on the board! I'm not sure how she knew to treat me differently than my previous teachers, but she definitely had more patience. Maybe she saw that my homework was always right but my classwork wasn't and put the pieces together to work it out!"

This answer demonstrates a real insight into why a teacher treated you how they did, and what the result of it was. It also implies that you are a good independent learner (which is always a bonus to slip into an answer!). When you are discussing why a teacher has treated you a certain way, it is important not to consider any of your own assumptions to be fact. Remember, the interviewer is likely also an educator, and they may see that your assumptions which you have made out to be fact, are likely wrong. It is, however, important that you outline what your views on how they treated you are, as even just the fact you are considering the reasons behind teachers' actions is a great way to better understand yourself and how you work best.

Q49: What are your long-term plans in life?

This question is incredibly open, and doesn't need to be answered like a 'where do you see yourself in x years' question. You can answer this question entirely unrelatedly to academia and work if you like. If your goal in life is to own your own home and have a family, say that! The important thing is to ground it around how this degree will help you get there. It could be something as simple as the degree with unlock doors in the job market that you wouldn't normally have been able to enter, or it could be that the degree will teach you how to work hard and independently, which will help you achieve things in later life. Whatever angle you approach it from, it is a great idea to include a piece about your degree studies.

However, you want to be honest with these plans as a question as open as this is a perfect opportunity for you to discuss something memorable to the interviewer. Maybe you have always wanted to be a clown, so working a job which pays well will enable you to go to clown school at the weekends and learn! It doesn't really matter what it is, as long as it's honest. If you start talking about something because you think it will be memorable, rather than because it is the truth, the interviewer will likely see right through you, so don't!

It is totally fine to have 'boring' aspirations, everyone's life is their own! If your aspirations in life are somewhat mundane, make that part of the explanation!

"I know it seems pretty mundane, but what I'd really like is to have a house, family and a stable job by the time I am thirty. This degree will teach me the skills I need to do well in the working world, unlock access to a job that I will enjoy, and enable me to earn the money I need to own my own home."

It isn't the most personality-injected answer, but if the above answer is honest then it is totally fine to go down that route! Obviously, if you have an honest ambition that is a little more whacky then discuss it, but don't feel like you have to make something up to be memorable! Honesty is the best policy, but try to make a link between whatever you're discussing and your degree studies. It doesn't have to be forced if it really doesn't work, but ideally you want your long-term plans to be tied into your degree, to some extent!

Q50: If you had to name your three greatest strengths, what would you pick?

This is a very open question. Because of this, it would be best to make at least one of these skills something to do with your degree and another something very personal to you. Beyond that, the floor is yours! When answering, for each skill you should explain what that skills is, where it originated, and how is has/will be useful to you. When talking about how it will be useful, that's where the degree studies bit comes in! Below is an example of how to outline one of these three skills.

"One of my top skills is my ability to type very fast and very accurately. I started typing pretty young because my mum worked from home and I used to use her keyboard to type fake emails while she was on her lunchbreak. I had to touch-type to a degree because I wasn't tall enough to see over her desk! When I started school, I used to get into accidents a lot so spent a few terms in various casts. Whenever that happened, I had to do all of my schoolwork on a laptop. Since starting sixth form, I've done all of my work on my laptop and have really honed my typing skills. These will definitely come in handy when writing essays, as I can much more easily and accurately write down citations!"

This answer brings some personality as it describes the origin of the skills, from an amusing childhood story to current working conditions in sixth form. If you are lucky to have a skill with such an extensive back story, then absolutely discuss it, even if perhaps you wouldn't consider it one of your top three skills! The clearest way to explore these three skills is to tell them as three individual stories, if you outline the skills first and go into the stories after, it will be too easy to get muddled and lose track of where you are. It would be great if you had skills which spread across a variety of disciplines. For example, in addition to the skill explained above, you could have one which relates to your social skills (e.g., recognising when someone is upset, even if they're trying to hide it) and one which relates to your physical ability (e.g., your proficiency at a certain sport). Of course, it would be all too convenient if that were the case, so don't try to bend the truth too much to get it to fit this model. It is better to be honest in a question like this, providing your answers have some degree of interest and relation to your subject!

Q51: How much should you charge to wash all the windows in London?

This question is not looking for an exact answer; instead the interviewer is inviting you to take them through your thought process as you make an estimate. Ultimately the tutorial experience is all about reasoning through often ambiguous or tricky problems, and this is an opportunity to demonstrate that you can do this.

A standard applicant might estimate the total surface area of windows in London, the average surface of windows washed per hour, and the hourly labour costs of window washing and use these to provide an answer. What will set a **good candidate** apart from a standard one is the quality of reasoning behind the numbers they come to. In this specific question, you would want to recognise that residential and commercial buildings, flats, and houses all have different numbers and sizes of windows. You may also want to consider other factors, such as London being a distinctly urban area, and windows potentially needing to be washed on both sides. Remember, these are just some possible considerations; there are all sorts of factors you could bring into the discussion.

For example, let us assume that there are 8 million people in London, and the average household is 2.5 people. This would mean that there are about 3.2 million households in London. You might then assume that the average number of windows across all residential and commercial buildings works out at 7.5 windows per household, and that the average surface area is 80cm by 50cm. To account for washing windows on both sides, you would multiply by 2 to give you the total surface area. Multiplying various decimals live might seem a bit daunting; feel free to round numbers where appropriate (and explain to the examiners why you are doing this). So in this example, you would calculate 3 million x 8 x 0.8 x 0.5 x 2 which would be about 19.2 million square meters of window.

From there you could discuss per hour labour costs, and the estimated surface area of windows you could wash per hour. Again, nuance is the key to making your answer stand out. Factors you might want to consider include (but are not limited to): skill required in window washing, cost of materials, cost of living in London, competition within the London window washing market, or whether the labour market is seasonal. Introducing these considerations offers you the opportunity to show not only that you are logical and rigorous, but also creative. To conclude this example, let us say you assume a wage of 10 pounds per hour, and 50 square meters of window per hour. This would give you a total cost of 3.84 million pounds.

A **weak answer** may have a very similar structure to a strong answer but lack the justification for numbers chosen. Other pitfalls to avoid include making simple calculation errors, and failing to use common sense when estimating numbers. For example by assuming that a population of 8 million people in London means that there are 8 million households. Avoid the temptation to be funny (e.g. answering "I have better things to do than wash windows"); this will not go down well.

Q52: How many piano tuners are there in Europe?

Although questions like this might seem initially daunting, the goal here is not to accurately estimate the number of piano tuners in Europe but rather to demonstrate clear, well explained reasoning.

In other words, a **good applicant** will offer sensible numbers backed up by a brief explanation as to how they chose these figures. For example, you could estimate that there are 750 million people in Europe, about 2.5 people per household, and therefore a total of 300 million households. Then by assuming that something like 1 in 50 households have a piano, you would estimate the number of pianos in Europe as around 6 million. Factors to consider when selecting these numbers could include how popular an instrument the piano is, or the cost of a piano. From there you could ascertain the number of piano tuners by dividing the average number of times people need their pianos tuned in a year by the number of pianos a piano tuner is able to tune in a year. When creating these numbers you could consider factors such as how long it takes to tune a piano, or how many days a year a piano tuner works (these are just a few examples, feel free to introduce your own ideas). For example, you could estimate that it takes a piano tuner 2 hours to tune a piano and they work about 8 hours a day, five days a week, for 50 weeks a year. This would amount to 1000 pianos per tuner per year. So, to carry out 5 million piano tunings you would need about 5000 piano tuners in Europe. Great answers could also introduce interesting considerations such as the potential impact of the increasing popularity of electric keyboards, and whether technological changes have led to an oversupply of trained piano tuners. Answers that contain deeper exploration like this help a candidate by showing nuanced, creative and forward-looking thinking.

A **poor applicant** will be thrown by the ambiguity of this kind of question and may just guess a number, or fail to use common sense or basic general knowledge; e.g. not offering even a rough idea of the population of Europe, or merely asserting the number of pianos tuned per year rather than estimating it logically. More generally, students should avoid the temptation to waffle when uncertain. What differentiates a weak from a strong answer, at least in part, is that the strong candidate will adopt a systematic and deductive approach to answering the question.

Q53: India introduces a new population control policy to address the gender imbalance. If a couple has a girl, they may have another child. If they have a boy, they can't have any more children. What would be the new ratio of boys to girls?

Obviously, the nature of this answer may vary substantially between applicants – a political scientist and a mathematician are likely to give very different answers. However, the essential thing is to be able to clarify and justify the assumptions that you are making when you answer this question.

For example, a **good quantitative candidate** might decide to discount any parental preference for one gender or the other, and assume that there is perfect compliance with the policy. From there, the candidate would note that every birth has a 50% independent probability of resulting in a girl and a 50% independent probability of resulting in a boy. This would mean that half of all families stop at one child, and the rest go on to have another child which also has a 50% chance of being a girl. Putting aside practical considerations, this process could repeat infinitely - although the probability of an unbroken chain of girls converges towards zero. The big thing to note here is that with each pregnancy the probability resets to 50/50. However, even when offering a quantitative answer the candidate should still acknowledge practical limitations (e.g. having infinite children is not possible).

More broadly, a **weaker answer** is likely to contain some of these elements but fail to identify key assumptions, or make implausible assumptions (e.g. parents having infinite numbers of children). Candidates who choose to use examples should also be wary of relying on anecdote rather than reasoning. For example, a weaker answer may use the example of China to discuss the effects of birth control policies on sex ratios, but simply argue that because sex ratios remain imbalanced in China they will do the same in India; it would be more useful to explore the similarities and differences between the two countries and their policy environment, rather than making a blanket correlation.

Q54: Why are manhole covers round?

As with many of the more unusual questions you may be asked, the key here is not to find the answer, but rather to demonstrate the ability to engage with ambiguous questions and reason logically. The key advice for questions such as this is to always try to tackle the question head on, engage with the hypothetical, and ask yourself why this specific question is being asked. This should hopefully help you to avoid the sort of woolly and non-committal answers that questions such as this often provoke.

A **strong candidate** would focus on the core of this question: what is distinctive about the circular shape (as opposed to, say, a square)? A good candidate will also avoid the trap of getting hung-up on the empirical question of whether all manhole covers are round – there is no need to go beyond an acknowledgement of this doubt. Focusing instead on the unique features of circles would allow the candidate time to offer a range of explanations as to why manhole might be round. Possible explanations could be that you do not need to worry about the orientation of a circle when replacing it back on to the hole, circles can be rolled which is useful since a manhole cover is usually heavy and made out of metal, or that round manhole covers are less likely to fall down the manhole. A great candidate will be able to specifically link this answer back to the purpose of a manhole. For example, the cover being easy to roll is likely to be important if you only have one person working on the manhole, or when a manhole is deep and so preventing things (people, or the cover) falling down the hole is very important.

A **weak answer** could take several forms. Candidates who attempt to debate whether manholes are all round, are unlikely to meet with much success. Although under certain circumstances disagreeing with the premise of a question can be a fruitful tactic, this rarely tends to be the case when the premise is a factual claim. Other weak approaches include offering a vague answer such as `tradition` or `culture`. Answers such as this one fail to engage with the core of the question; a good warning sign is that your answer could apply to a broad range of other questions. If this is the case, your answer is probably lacking in specificity.

Q55: How many times per day does a clock's hand overlap?

There many ways of getting the answer other than the one provided below; however, more important than the specific method is walking through the steps in your reasoning clearly and logically. This does not just demonstrate your thinking process to the interviewer, but will also help you to avoid making silly mistakes by jumping to an answer too quickly. If you find it hard to structure your thoughts in your head, consider taking a minute to write down your thought process on a piece of paper.

A **good answer:** On a 12-hour clock face the hour hand completes two full circles in a day, and the minute hand does a full rotation every hour; i.e. 24 rotations in a day. Having established these facts, one approach is to visualise the first time the two hands cross. If you start from midnight with the hands in the same position you would need to wait for at least one full rotation before they intersect. Since the hour hand is moving from midnight to 1am the intersection would be at roughly 1:05 (it would actually be a bit later since the hour hand would actually be at the 1 when the minute was at the 12). Now we know that the two hands cross at approximately 1.05 we can visualize the next overlap which would be when the hour hand is at about 2 and the minute hand is at about 10 minutes past (again the numbers are not quite exact). What you might notice here is that the overlaps happen at about 65 minutes intervals. There are 14400 minutes in a day (60 x 24), so if you divide 14400 by 65 you get a little over 22. Therefore the total number of overlaps would be 22.

As noted above, a **weak answer** may occur due to simple calculation error or trying to jump to the answer too quickly. For example: "The minute hand goes around the clock 24 times in a day, so it presumably crosses the minute hand once each time. So that would be 24." Many candidates may slip up on this question by choosing a seemingly obvious answer. The larger lesson to draw from this is that if a solution seems obvious, ask yourself whether it is likely that the interviewer would get any value from seeing you solve this problem. Not only the content, but also the brevity may be a warning sign that your answer is on the wrong track.

Q56: You are given 7 identical balls and another ball that looks the same as the others but is heavier than them. You can use a balance only two times. How would you identify which is the heavy ball?

Although questions like this may seem somewhat intimidating the best way to approach them is to start by slowly working step by step. You do not necessarily have to start with the correct method, but try to work towards it and rule out less useful approaches as you go.

A good candidate might start by noting that they do not know how much heavier the heavy ball is. From this information they can deduce that placing 3 balls on one side of the scale and 4 balls on the other may not give us precise enough information. Instead, for a more accurate approach we must start by placing an equal number of items on each side. If one places three balls on each side, then whichever side is heavier must include the heavy ball. However, if the balance is equal then the heavy ball must be the ball that was not placed on the scale. From here a candidate could deduce that either they had solved the problem, or they would need to repeat the experiment with the three balls on the heavy side of the balance. In this instance, the candidate would compare two of the balls from the heavier side and set the third ball aside. If either of the two balls on the balance was heavier we would have our answer, or if they were equal, the remaining ball that the candidate had set aside would be the heavier ball.

By contrast, **a weaker candidate** may use a process of trial and error instead of taking a step back, drawing conclusions from their thinking and using these new conclusions to inform their next move. Note that not all strong candidates will immediately come to the solution; the difference between the strong and the weak candidate is that a strong candidate will be able to course-correct as they go and spot the nature of their error, whereas a weak candidate may not be able to identify where they made a mistake.

Q57: What is your favourite number?

This question is a great opportunity for you to demonstrate enthusiasm for your chosen subject. For example, as a mathematician you may find a specific number theoretically interesting, as a historian you could pick a specific date, or as a biologist you might pick a number that represents an interesting phenomenon in the natural world (e.g. rate of bacterial reproduction). When answering the question, take care to pick something that you genuinely find interesting and can talk about at length, rather than something you think will sound impressive. Make sure the interviewer remembers you for the whole content of and justification for your answer, not just the opening line.

Although personal stories are unlikely to harm you, choosing your grandmother's birthday, a football player's jersey number or the numbers you always pick for the lottery is unlikely to strengthen your application. The important thing to remember when confronted with an unexpected question is to take a step back and think about how you can direct the conversation to something that will bolster your case for admission.

Finally, although it is important to draw in interesting content about your subject, a good candidate will also answer the question. A **weaker answer** might use the answer as a springboard to offer a prepared answer on an unrelated topic. For example, cite a historical date and then simply talk about their interest in that historical period. By contrast a **strong answer** might talk about the role numbers play in memory, or the importance of quantification in history. These answers are stronger because they focus on the core of the question and justify why the number is a relevant feature of the answer, rather than the number being an afterthought. Directly engaging with the question is important as it shows that you are responding authentically and in the moment, rather than seeming like a poor listener or an overprepared candidate.

Q58: Who am I? (Always read up on your interviewers!)

This is a good opportunity for a candidate to demonstrate they have thought about their college choice and know who the tutors in their subject area are; this is a chance to show that you are thoughtful and engaged with your chosen degree subject.

Good answer: 'You are Professor X, you work in the field of [biomedical science, economics, etc]. I think more specifically you work in the subfield of [human anatomy/microeconomics] and some of your research looks at [cerebral cortical development/auction theory]. I was really excited about applying to this college because, as I mentioned in my personal statement, I am particularly interested in [the role of cortical development in conditions such as dyslexia/the application of auction theory to public goods tenders].'

This is a good answer because it shows that the candidate has serious academic reasons for applying to a college, and has begun to develop interests within their subject area. Of course, this is contingent on these interests being real. Do not bring up research if you do not understand it; this is likely to lead to embarrassment! There are other ways to answer this question. For example, a tutor might state on their college webpage that they love working with undergraduates, or you may have seen them give an inspiring talk at an Open Day. These are also valid things to bring up about a tutor, as they have chosen to put this information in the public domain.

A **weak answer** could go in a lot of different directions. For example, the student might attempt to move in an excessively abstract direction (e.g. what is the nature of identity?) - this might be OK if you are in a philosophy interview, but less so for subjects like maths. Alternatively, the student may simply not know who the interviewer is. You will typically be interviewed by fellows at the college, so you should have the opportunity to have a look at their research. Additionally, you are normally told who your interviewers will be prior to the interview, which should give you an opportunity to look them up.

Q59: Is there any question that you wished we had asked you?

This question is a great chance to highlight an aspect of your application that you would like to talk about. For example, you may have written about a specific book on your personal statement that you think you can speak about further in an interesting manner, or you might have written an extended essay which demonstrates your interest in and understanding of a specific subject. Thanking the interviewers and expressing enthusiasm about the content can also be a nice touch. However, it is inadvisable to simply state your desire to go to Oxbridge, or launch into abstract declarations of your love for the subject. These should be demonstrated through actions not words; over the top displays of emotion are more likely to make an interviewer uncomfortable than convince them to admit you.

More commonly, however, what will differentiate a strong from a weak answer is not the topic but rather the manner in which you talk about it. For example, a **strong answer** should highlight an aspect of your application in a concise manner that directly underscores your commitment to the subject and shows intellectual maturity. However, you do need to make the case as to why you want to discuss this; it should not come across as simply a desire to introduce impressive things you have done. Ways to avoid this include explaining why a given activity demonstrates your curiosity about your subject, or perhaps an interest in the process of academic research.

A **weaker answer** could come in many different forms. Any answer that strays into boasting or flattery is unlikely to make a favourable impression. If you genuinely do not have any topics you would like to discuss it is fine to admit to this; interviewers know that the interview experience can be stressful and not all candidates (even strong ones) will relish the prospect of further interview questions!

Q60: What are you looking forward to the least at this college?

This is a question where you can be honest to a certain extent, but must remain balanced. **Poor answers** are likely to fall into one of two extremes; the 'fake problem' or the 'too blunt'. Interviewers are unlikely to believe the candidate who claims that they are least looking forward to a choice of modules because they wish they could choose everything (is that really the worst possible thing you could think of?). As a result, this attempt to avoid admitting to any negative or undesirable opinion risks coming off as insincere. However, veering too far in the opposite direction is also inadvisable. Saying you are worried about the workload before you have even arrived is likely to raise red flags and make interviewers wonder whether you will be able to cope with the pace of Oxbridge.

By contrast a **good answer** will strike a balance between sincerity and oversharing by stating a genuine concern - but ideally one that does not relate to academic concerns. For example, you could quite reasonably express concerns about financial stability, being able to find a common cultural community, or other similar considerations. If these are genuine concerns, they are things a college will be interested in knowing so that they can try to help solve them. If you are struggling to find an appropriate concern, while not ideal it is OK to say that you will miss your cat, home cooking, or that you are mostly very excited about going to university and so do not yet have anything you are very worried about.

Ultimately, this sort of question serves two functions for interviewers: it helps them to decide whether students are applying for the right reasons (academic work not college balls), but also to make sure that they are aware of applicants concerns. Colleges really do want to make themselves accessible and friendly places, so this is a time when it can be appropriate to raise a concern or question that may have been bothering you.

Q61: Who has had the largest influence on your life?

Questions such as these should be answered in a way that is first and foremost plausible, and secondly makes the case for you as a candidate. Ways you can make that case include demonstrating that your interest in your chose subject is deep and long-standing (i.e. you didn't apply on a whim and you have specific subject interests).

Weak answers may come from candidates too eager to impress interviewers with their passion for their subject. Very few people are likely to believe that Marie Curie has had more influence on your life than a family member, or caregiver. It is important to remember that seeming genuine is just as important as seeming intelligent (if not more so). Other ways candidates can provide weak answers include being too laconic, or unreflective. Failing to relate the answer to your current subject interests, while not something that is likely to be penalised, might be a bit of a missed opportunity.

Explanation is the key to a **good answer**. For example, you might quite plausibly be able to say that your mum has been the biggest influence on your life, briefly discuss non-academic ways in which she has influenced you and then discuss how she has had a role in your intellectual development. Maybe she encountered problems when finding work that made you want to become an economist to better understand the labour market. Perhaps at a certain point she stopped being able to answer your questions about the world, and as a result you wanted to become a biologist. Ultimately, the connection you make will depend on both your subject and your chosen person. Of course, sometimes a connection to your degree will not be obvious, and that is fine. It is better to have a natural seeming answer than forcing a subject matter connection where none exists, and running the risk of seeming disingenuous.

Q62: If you were me, would you let yourself in?

Although some people might feel a temptation to answer 'no' to stand out, this is not the time for being wacky. Instead, treat this as an opportunity to advocate for yourself while also addressing any perceived weaknesses you might have. Each candidate will vary in the traits that make them distinctive, so answers will differ substantially between candidates. However, a **strong candidate** should start by considering qualities that Oxbridge might look for in a candidate, and then assess themselves against this framework. Not only does this directly answer the question, but also demonstrates to the interviewer that the candidate is a structured and rigorous thinker.

For example, you might start by defining a 'good' candidate as having both a deep interest in their subject, and academic aptitude. You might then illustrate your interest in your subject by referring to your personal statement and extra-curriculars. This could include addressing any weakness (e.g. mixed GCSE results) with reference to a mitigating or balancing factor (e.g. a strong focus on science subjects, and strong predicted A-levels). Any suggestion that a weakness is either acceptable or irrelevant should be backed up by a plausible explanation; if you believe that an explanation will simply sound like an excuse, it may be better to not raise it at all.

A **poor candidate** may have woolly reasoning or be unable to explain what makes them distinctive - many candidates will have excellent marks and a good personal statement. It is also inadvisable to speak negatively about other candidates (even in broad brush terms). For example, I am X unlike all of Y who are the same. You can make points about your own distinctiveness without coming across as mean-spirited or negative. Remember that these interviewers will have to teach you; they do not just want to know you are clever, they also want to know that working together will be an enjoyable experience.

Q63: What do you think my favourite colour is? Why do you say that?

Although many questions offer the opportunity to demonstrate your interest in your subject, in certain circumstances you may have trouble doing so naturally. Again, answering the question and demonstrating good listening skills is key. In situations such as these, rather than offering a tangential and canned answer, think of critical thinking strengths you can highlight through your answer. In this instance, good deductive reasoning and clear communication can help you demonstrate to your interviewer that you are a clear and logical student who will fare well in tutorials.

A **good answer** may discuss how a favourite colour might influence someone's clothing or room decoration choices. This would not be simple reasoning, such as "people will wear their favourite colour", but would introduce nuance by considering limitations to the evidence that they are using. For example, if you really like bright pink or bright green you might not wear that colour in a professional setting, or just limit it to somewhere inconspicuous such as a tie, or a pair of socks. Importantly, although a good answer will consider limitations to reasoning it *should* come to a conclusion. A candidate who twists themselves in knots of uncertainty will come across as a messy thinker who is not able to weigh competing pieces of evidence. By all means acknowledge weaknesses in your logic or contradictory evidence, but you should offer a guess.

A **weak answer** might suffer from a lack of nuance; or conversely a candidate may be so aware of the limitations of their reasoning that they offer a long-winded reply that ultimately comes to no conclusion. Other pitfalls include coming across as combative or annoyed by a seemingly irrelevant question. Although the interview experience can be stressful, being polite and upbeat is key; these are people you will have to work with.

Q64: What is a lie? How do I know what you just said isn't a lie?

In questions that ask you to offer definitions of complex concepts, a great way to start is by using examples to explore your initial intuition. Interviewers are unlikely to expect you to have a ready-made definition; many of these concepts are the subject of intense academic debate! What *is* important, however, is showing that you are a creative thinker who can course-correct and explore their own thinking in a structured manner.

For example, a **strong candidate** might start with a definition such as "a lie is a statement that is knowingly false", and then use specific examples to test whether this definition fits across a range of contexts. For example, what does it mean to lie to oneself? What is the role of intent in the definition of lying? Are 'white lies' still lies? These are just a few examples of questions a candidate might raise, and there are no definitive right or wrong answers. Instead, the important feature of a good answer is that a candidate can navigate from the intellectually abstract definition to a concrete situation with fluency, demonstrating both strong conceptual thinking and an ability to drive their own intellectual process. The use of examples is a great way to do this because it allows you to ground your answer in everyday experience and may help you to tease out weaknesses or contradictions in your thinking. Again, coming to a conclusion (or at least a specific definition) is critical to a good answer. You can certainly acknowledge weaknesses or uncertainties, but a good candidate should be able to weigh evidence and come down on a side.

By contrast, a **weaker candidate** is likely to be less reflective about the quality of their own answer, and perhaps rush to a conclusion (or be unwilling to come to one at all). One mistake that candidates often make is thinking that an interview is a debate; that they are obliged to stick to and defend their original statements. In fact, it is often a great idea to let your position evolve if you change your mind. Tutors are looking for people who are open-minded and intellectually flexible.

Q65: If you could keep objects from the present for the future, what would they be?

Rather than taking this as a whimsical or warm up question, use this as an opportunity to highlight your passion for your subject. This will naturally vary from candidate to candidate, but the broad lesson is that even seemingly off the wall questions can be used to strengthen your case for admission.

A **good answer** from an historian might, for example, highlight their thoughts about the importance of sources to future generations of historians. A biologist may be interested in species preservation and want to keep a patch of the Amazon. In instances where material objects might be less relevant to your subject (e.g. as an economist, or a theoretical physicist), you could show creativity by suggesting an item emblematic of a phenomenon you find interesting (e.g. promotional material from the sharing economy, or the computer used to carry out complex calculations).

A weaker answer could take many different forms, but failing to relate your answer to your subject or poorly justifying your choice are common errors. Many weak answers use the same examples as stronger ones, but simply fail to fully explain why they selected the item. For example, a biologist simply saying "I would preserve a tree in the Amazon because I think that the biodiversity in underexplored areas of the rainforest is enormous, and I think deforestation might eradicate our chances to access this knowledge" does not fully demonstrate that the candidate understands what they are talking about. Their answer remains very general and does not specify what sort of information they are concerned about preserving. A candidate in this position could easily strengthen their answer by drawing on examples of findings they have read about, thus demonstrating that their example is not a vague concern about the environment but rooted in specific knowledge indicative of a deep curiosity about their subject.

Q66: What is more important – art or science?

As with many abstract questions, a **good answer** will offer clear reasoning, an acknowledgement of alternative positions, and an explicit conclusion. For example, you may believe that *generally speaking* science is more important than art because science is central to material improvements in people's well-being. You might then acknowledge some weaknesses in this position, e.g. that this is not true of all science (certain forms of pure mathematics have no known practical application), or that art can be critical to social or moral progress. Finally, do offer a rebuttal (e.g. physical life is the basis of all other values and so although art is important, medical advances are necessary to enjoy art). These are just a few examples of arguments that could be raised, and a compelling case could be made on either side.

A **weaker answer** may offer the same general reasoning as the strong answer, but simply fail to offer much justification. Another common trap is listing the advantages and disadvantages of both disciplines but failing to explain how you weigh these different considerations. This is a question that may arouse strong feelings in many candidates who want to demonstrate their interest in their chosen subject; however, you should be careful about coming across as brow beating, or arrogant. Even if you – as a scientist – believe that art can only exist because of scientific progress, there are ways to explain this view without seeming dismissive of something that many others value enormously. The same applies to humanities students who believe that life only has meaning due to art – beware of sounding pretentious! Once again, always remember that your interviewer may tutor you in the future, so coming across as friendly and open-minded is just as important as seeming clever. Launching into a tirade is more likely to make you seem unreflective than passionate.

Q67: If you could have one superpower, which one would it be? Why?

Seemingly random questions can often be used as an opportunity to talk about your interest in your subject. One way of answering this question would be to think of a problem that you face in your field, and select a superpower that would help you resolve it. Obviously, omniscience might do this, but probably also makes for a less interesting answer.

As with other questions of this variety, what will differentiate a good answer from a weak answer is not the topic chosen, but rather the explanation given. For example, a historian could talk about their desire to time travel; but what would distinguish a good answer from a weak or commonplace one would be the justification. For example, a **weaker candidate** might simply say "I am interested in Napoleonic history so I would love to be able to observe the Battle of Waterloo". While the candidate may talk specifically what they would like to see and demonstrate strong understanding of Napoleonic history, enthusiasm for historical facts is not the same as showing a scholarly approach.

By contrast, a **strong candidate** might discuss their desire to go to a specific period and then relate this to an interest in collecting oral history sources. In an answer such this, the student not only explains their reasoning and relates it to a specific personal interest, but they also display good knowledge of the problems scholars of their subject might face. All of this suggests a mature thinker who would do well at university.

Although a time travelling historian might seem like an obvious example, similar answers can come from a variety of disciplines. A physicist might want to be able to observe unobservable events, a biologist might want eyes with the power of microscopes. Ultimately this sort of question is very open to interpretation and the strength of the answer will lie in the justification.

Q68: Would you ever go on a one-way trip to Mars? Why/why not?

As ever, you should treat every question as an opportunity to highlight why you would be a good candidate for admission. Even questions such as this, which may appear to be utterly random, can often be related back to your chosen subject. However, it is also fine to inject human concerns into your answers; it is always important for your reply to seem natural.

For example, a **good answer** from a biologist might talk about their desire to know more about microbial life on Mars, and their interest in the findings of the Mars Curiosity Rover, but ultimately conclude that they would rather rely on earth-based study than abandon their family. The student expresses enthusiasm for their subject, but also sets out quite reasonable limits on what they are willing to sacrifice for science. This honesty may come across as more credible than the candidate who claims that they would be willing to abandon their family and friends. A word to the wise: if you do raise specific examples (e.g. microbial life) then be certain that you can talk about them in more depth if probed. For non-STEM candidates, a clear relationship to your subject may be harder to draw; but creative thinking should allow you to find one. For example, historians might draw parallels with prior explorers of the globe, and philosophers could establish an ethical framework for evaluating such a choice. However, even if you cannot think of a link to your subject, remember to offer clear reasoning and a conclusion.

A **weak answer** could fall into any of the pitfalls mentioned above. Although it is fine to answer that one would indeed take a one-way trip, making sweeping claims such as "I love physics so much I would abandon my family and live alone on Mars" may ring somewhat hollow. Other weak answers may simply fail to grasp the opportunity to relate their thinking back to their subject. While this is unlikely to actively harm the your chances, it would be a missed opportunity.

Q69: Does human nature change?

Questions which ask candidates to discuss abstract concepts are a great opportunity to demonstrate to your interviewer that you are a structured thinker, who can engage with high level concepts and not get muddled. To answer this question well, the candidate needs to explore what people mean by the term 'human nature'. The candidate may also want to explore what is meant by the term 'change', and under what circumstances their answer might vary.

A **good candidate** might, for example, discuss whether the use of the term 'nature' implies some unchanging essence. There are a variety of strategies a candidate could adopt to do this effectively, including looking at examples of when people use the term 'human nature' and what they tend to be explaining when they do this. Alternatively, the candidate may want to provide a direct definition of human nature (e.g. the basic motivations of all homo sapiens). Strong candidates will also seek to define the parameters of their answer. Rather than simply providing a yes or no conclusion to their answer the candidate may offer a qualified response, e.g. "Yes, human nature can change over time, but a single individual cannot change their nature". While this is just an example, answers such as these show to the interviewer that the candidate has thought deeply about their answer and is able to generate a rigorous conceptual framework on the fly.

Weaker answers are likely to fall into one of a few different traps. Some candidates mistake conversations such as these for a debate and try to defend their instinctive initial answer; however, this can often come across as intellectual inflexibility, or arrogance. Showing willingness to engage with new ideas and revise your own when confronted with (reasonable) criticism can be a strength. Other candidates struggle with the lack of structure provided by this question and will throw out a range of possible considerations but be unable to draw them together into any coherent answer. Taking a minute before answering the question to jot down some thoughts can be a good way to give your answer more structure.

Q70: Define 'success' in one sentence.

This question, like many of the more abstract questions asked, is an opportunity for the candidate to showcase the quality of their thinking when confronted with an unfamiliar topic. Beyond simply showing clear and logical reasoning, candidates can also excel by using this question as an opportunity to emphasise their passion for their subject through their choice of examples.

For example, **a good candidate** might start with an initial definition that is further refined as they reason out loud. One way to do this would be work through a few examples to test whether the definition of success they came up with holds true in each case. An answer would be enhanced if the examples the candidate chooses not only draw on their subject matter expertise, but are also a little unusual. For example, an art historian could, of course, discuss whether Van Gogh (who died in penury) can be considered a success; but this is an example even a non-subject specialist might come up with. By contrast, selecting an artist from a period the candidate mentioned in their personal statement would allow them to demonstrate that their interest has real depth to it.

As with many with many of these abstract questions, a **weak answer** to this question is likely to be caused by a lack of structure, or under-explanation. A good answer and a weak answer may start off with the same definition; but where the quality of the answers will diverge is in the explanation of how a candidate came to that answer. A weaker candidate may offer examples of success as evidence, whereas the good candidate will use examples to pick out specific features of what could and could not be called success. Returning to the Van Gogh example, the strong candidate might point to the tension between the lack of recognition during his lifetime and his subsequent acclaim, and then examine whether or not we would call him a success if he had been famous during his lifetime and then forgotten. By contrast, the weaker candidate's exploration may be limited to noting that 'success can happen outside of your lifetime'.

Q71: Is there such a thing as truth?

Applicants can adopt one of two strategies to answer this question well. As ever, students can draw examples from their own subject to illustrate their answer; for example, mathematicians might want to talk about proofs, and historians might want to talk about source reliability. Alternatively, students can take this as an opportunity to simply show clear reasoning, and good verbal expression. The best applicants may be able to combine these two approaches.

A **good candidate** might start with a simple answer that they explicitly state they plan to refine. An example of such an answer would be "I think there is such a thing as truth, and I will define truth as a statement that describes a situation that exists or has existed in the world". From there, the candidate might use situations which appear to be truthful but do not cohere with this definition to examine whether it is possible to come to a meaningful definition of truth. For example, they might examine whether statements which are mildly inaccurate can be called truth and whether it is possible to make truly accurate statements (e.g. can we say that 'the cat jumped on the table five minutes ago' is a lie, if the cat jumped on the table 6 minutes ago?). Good candidates will also note that certain domains might have 'truth' and others might not. For example, do moral or aesthetic statements have truth value?

A **weaker applicant** is likely to offer a less thoughtful answer. The weakest answers are likely to be characterised by brevity: "Yes, because I can say that this chair is here, and it is. That's a true statement". Although you may believe this to be true, it is always worth fleshing an answer out by exploring where you could be wrong. Less obviously weak answers are likely to suffer from a lack of structure. It is very possible for a candidate to raise a few interesting thoughts but fail to explore them comprehensively or organise them well. While intellectual promise is helpful, without clear explanation a candidate's answer may simply be interpreted as scattershot.

Q72: You are shrunk down so you're the size of a matchstick and then put into a blender with metal blades. It is about to be turned on – what do you do?

This question can be used to demonstrate all sorts of different skills, from creativity to analytical thinking, and could even show how you are able to apply subject knowledge to an unusual problem. The physicists, biologists, and engineers out there may want to ask clarifying questions about the scenario to gain more information, such as the density of the shrunken human body. If you can explain why these questions are relevant and how they influence your answer, then ask away – it is often an excellent way to engage.

For those for whom there may be no obvious subject connection, a **good candidate** could simply work through the problem by breaking it down into component pieces. As with any non-traditional question there is no single correct way of doing this. For example, certain candidates might identify that there are two solutions: break the machine or avoid the blades. They could then discuss which of these two solutions would be more likely to succeed and then select that solution. Other equally successful candidates might consider whether someone is trying to blend them intentionally - and if not, how someone so small might be able to attract the attention of the person about to turn on the blender. Candidates are, of course, also expected to show basic common sense; just because a situation is fantastical does not mean that they can posit absurd solutions. Candidates should try to consider realistic features such as the centrifugal force of the blades, or strength of the machine relative to someone the size of a matchstick.

Weaker candidates are less likely to be let down by the content of their answers, than by the lack of enthusiasm, intellectual curiosity, or flexibility that they demonstrate. Note that even the good candidate may not find a satisfying solution to this (rather strange) problem; but what they will do is explore a variety of ideas, and demonstrate the ability to evaluate their own thought process while remaining engaged with the interview.

BIOLOGY & MEDICINE

There is a large degree of overlap between the biological sciences and Medicine at Oxbridge. Medical interviews at Oxbridge are likely to focus on the human side of biology (physiology, pathology, pharmacology etc). One of the medical interviews maybe a 'general' one- similar in style to the classical medical interviews (with questions like *"how do you deal with stress?"* etc). This latter style of interview is beyond the confines of this book. The advice that follows is applicable to both biology and medicine applicants due to their similarity.

In general, you'll be **tackling a large question with many smaller sub-questions** to guide the answer from the start to a conclusion. The main question may seem difficult, impossible or random at first, but take a deep breath and start discussing different ideas that you have for breaking the question down into manageable pieces.

The questions are designed to be difficult to give you the chance to **show your full intellectual potential**. The interviewers will help guide you to the right idea provided you work with them and offer ideas for them to steer you along with. This is your chance to show your creativity, analytical skills, intellectual flexibility, problem-solving skills, and your go-getter attitude. Don't waste it by letting your nerves overtake or from a fear of messing up or looking stupid.

MEDICAL ETHICS

Medical applicants are commonly asked medical ethics questions, so it's well worth knowing the basics. Whilst there are huge ethical textbooks available— you only need to be familiar with the basic principles for the purposes of your interview. **These principles can be applied to all cases** regardless what the social/ethnic background the healthcare professional or patient is from. The principles are:

Beneficence: The wellbeing of the patient should be the doctor's first priority. In medicine this means that one must act in the patient's best interests to ensure the best outcome is achieved for them i.e. 'Do Good'.

Non-Maleficence: This is the principle of avoiding harm to the patient (i.e. Do no harm). There can be a danger that in a willingness to treat, doctors can sometimes cause more harm to the patient than good. This can especially be the case with major interventions, such as chemotherapy or surgery. Where a course of action has both potential harms and potential benefits, non-maleficence must be balanced against beneficence.

Autonomy: The patient has the right to determine their own health care. This, therefore, requires the doctor to be a good communicator so that the patient is sufficiently informed to make their own decisions. 'Informed consent' is thus a vital precursor to any treatment. A doctor must respect a patient's refusal of treatment even if they think it is not the correct choice. Note that patients cannot <u>demand</u> treatment – only refuse it, e.g. an alcoholic patient can refuse rehabilitation but cannot demand a liver transplant.

There are many situations where the application of autonomy can be quite complex, for example:

- **Treating Children**: Consent is required from the parents, although the autonomy of the child is taken into account increasingly as they get older.
- **Treating adults without the capacity** to make important decisions. The first challenge with this is in assessing whether or not a patient has the capacity to make the decisions. Just because a patient has a mental illness does not necessarily mean that they lack the capacity to make decisions about their health care. Where patients do lack capacity, the power to make decisions is transferred to the next of kin (or Legal Power of Attorney, if one has been set up).

Justice: This principle deals with the fair distribution and allocation of healthcare resources for the population.

Consent: This is an extension of Autonomy- patients must agree to a procedure or intervention. For consent to be valid, it must be **voluntary informed consent.** This means that the patient must have sufficient mental capacity to make the decision and must be presented with all the relevant information (benefits, side effects and the likely complications) in a way they can understand.

Confidentiality: Patients expect that the information they reveal to doctors will be kept private- this is a key component in maintaining the trust between patients and doctors.

You must ensure that patient details are kept confidential. Confidentiality can be broken if you suspect that a patient is a risk to themselves or to others e.g. Terrorism, suicides.

Ensure that you don't immediately give an answer – consider both sides of the argument (pros and cons) and discuss them in detail before arriving at a balanced conclusion.

WORKED QUESTIONS

Below are a few examples of how to start breaking down an interview question, complete with model answers.

Q1: Why do we see colour blindness in women less than men?

[Extremely clear-headed] <u>Applicant:</u> *Well, I know that women are much less likely to be colour-blind than men. Why don't I start by defining colour-blindness and working out why there is a gender difference using Mendelian inheritance, and then think about mechanisms of colour-blindness which may not be accounted for in this method. I noticed you specified females in relation to males, so I'm going to suggest that whatever <u>this mechanism is, it is sex-dependent.</u>*

Now, being this clear-headed is unlikely to happen when put on the spot, unless you practice a lot, but it shows that the question can be broken down into sub-parts, which can be dealt with in turn. At this point, the interviewer can give feedback if this seems like a good start and help make any modifications if necessary. The applicant would realise that colour-blindness is inherited on the X-chromosome and the second female X-chromosome may help compensate. Although a single defective X-chromosome would lead to colour-blindness, having two defective X-chromosomes does not necessarily mean that a woman would be colour-blind as the defects might be opposites and therefore cancel each other to lead to normal colour vision. The details are unimportant, but the general idea of <u>breaking down the question into manageable parts is important.</u>

The interviewer is not looking for a colour-blindness expert, but someone who can problem-solve in the face of new ideas. Note that this is a question about Proximate Causes in disguise; although the question begins with 'Why', it is actually asking 'how' or which mechanism is causing this discrepancy.

A <u>poor applicant</u> may take a number of approaches unlikely to impress the interviewer. The first and most obvious of these is to say, "We never learned about colour-blindness in school" and make no attempt to move forward from this. The applicants who have done this only make it worse for themselves by resisting prompting as the interviewer attempts to pull an answer from them, saying "fine, but I'm not going to know the answer because I don't know anything about this", or an equally unenthusiastic and uncooperative response. Another approach which is unhelpful in the interview is the 'brain dump', where instead of engaging with the question, the applicant attempts to impress or distract with an assortment of related facts: "Colour-blindness mainly affects men. You can be completely colour-blind or red-green colour-blind. Many animals are colour-blind, but some also see a greater number of colours." Having gotten off to this start isn't as impressive as a more reasoned response, but the interview can be salvaged by taking the interviewer's feedback on-board. Many of these facts could start a productive discussion which leads to the answer if the applicant listens and takes hints and suggestions from the interviewer.

Q2: Do you think we have an ethical obligation to stop climate change?

This is a question about Ethics. To answer a question like this, the important thing is not to have a strong opinion that you defend to the death, but to be able to discuss the different viewpoints based on different understandings of right and wrong, and always with a sound understanding of the underlying issues- both scientific and humanitarian.

One way to break down this question would be to <u>consider whether an ethical obligation extends only to other humans or to other organisms</u> as well, and whether it applies in any situation or only when contributing to a situation that wouldn't occur naturally. Similarly, one could also discuss whether humans as a whole are obliged to halt global warming or just a select few members of the human race. Showing an ability to think flexibly about abstract concepts is always good, but don't forget to then argue for the different cases using knowledge of past and present climates and environments, as this is the subject-relevant part of the question.

For instance, as you are a scientist, don't waste time discussing if climate change is a reality – the scientific community has already reached a consensus. However, if you would like to argue against an ethical obligation instead, discuss the natural climate variations which have occurred on Earth in the past. Use probable climate change-driven events, like the Perma-Triassic extinction when 96% of species died out 250 million years ago, to argue that humans have no ethical obligation to save other species from anthropogenic extinction, because <u>even without human presence there are climate-driven extinctions.</u> Or argue the opposite, that despite past extreme environmental change being a reality, humanity is pushing the Earth further than it has ever sustained humans, and that we are obligated to do our part to leave a habitable Earth for people in other parts of the world and the future. Alternatively, argue completely that there can be no ethical obligation because everyone <u>contributes to the problem in their own way</u> and everyone will face the consequences. Or that only those who contribute more than they suffer are in the wrong for dumping their consequences onto others. Whichever argument you put forward, be sure to include scientific examples so that your discussion doesn't veer away from the question.

Remember that climate change is not the same as global warming and your discussion could include pollution (trash, toxins, chemicals, light and sound pollution, etc.), agriculture and monoculture, invasive species, hunting and fishing, deforestation and habitat fragmentation, or any of the other issues beyond the Greenhouse Effect which affect the environment.

Similarly, global warming is not just about fossil fuel use and carbon dioxide, but a range of gases and their effects on weather, ocean acidity, desertification, pathogen spread, etc. Show that you have a deeper understanding of these issues than you could get from skimming the headlines of the Daily Mail.

Q3: Why do we find DNA inside the nucleus, instead of mitochondria?

This is a question mainly about Ultimate Causes. While you could attempt to answer this by explaining proximate causes; **how** DNA is used and that it can't be in mitochondria, by giving reasons like "transcription occurs in the nucleus so it has to be there", you would be missing the important **why** part of this question. It is asking for an ultimate reason. In this case, for the evolutionary history which led mitochondria to have their own separate reproduction. Although **you are unlikely to know about this in detail**, it is important that you engage with this part of the question so that the interviewer can guide you.

Applicant: DNA can't be stored in the mitochondria because the mitochondria are genetically separate from the host cell. When the cell replicates its DNA and divides, the mitochondria separately replicate their own genetic material and reproduces to populate the new cell. The reason for the mitochondria having separate and distinct genetic material not identical to that of the host cell has been proposed to lie in the evolution of eukaryotes. The **Endosymbiotic Theory** suggests that cell organelles, particularly energy-producing chloroplasts and mitochondria, were originally separate prokaryotes that were engulfed by larger prokaryotes. They are believed to have begun a symbiotic relationship where perhaps the host cell receives energy and the mitochondria receive a safe environment for reproduction. As this symbiotic relationship evolved, the cells have exchanged some genetic material to coordinate their life-cycles and now cannot survive independently. This explains both the distinct genetic material of mitochondria and the double membrane which surrounds them in the cell – one the original prokaryotic membrane and one from being engulfed by the host. If they were originally a separate organism this explains why cell DNA cannot be stored there.

Q4: How would you determine the function of a human gene?

This is a question about the practical applications of genetics and experimental techniques – it is asking you to use your knowledge of genetics and research methods to come up with some practical ways of answering this. There are many ways you could answer this question, so take an approach that will allow you to use many examples which show off your knowledge, experience or extra reading about this subject.

If you only know about Mendelian genetics, you could suggest **searching the genome of relatives to a person known to have the gene** to see if those with the gene share traits. This would be a good time to mention a technique if you know it e.g. PCR. However, it may not be possible to isolate gene function this way because:

- The gene would need to be active
- Any trait it contributed to would need to be single locus to really see an effect
- It could produce a hidden condition that isn't apparent in a pedigree
- The gene could be essential and thus present in all relatives
- The sample size is so low that making spurious correlations is very likely
- This would only be a correlation study and not an experiment that determined cause and effect (experiments requiring human breeding are, at best, inconvenient)

If you are more familiar with genetics you may have other ideas; perhaps a cross-species survey looking for the gene in other species to judge its age and specificity to human life, or knock-out genetics with a closely related species possessing the gene to see if its presence is vital or has a direct effect.

The gene could be added to a bacterial genome using plasmids to see which protein is produced. No matter what your answer is, the important part of this question is to take a practical and self-critical approach which plays to your individual knowledge base.

A **poor applicant** would disregard that the question is asking for a practical solution and instead tell the interviewer about the general function of genes, or would ignore the specifics of the question- treating it as if it could be solved through Mendel's pea-flower approach. A poor applicant would not be self-critical and would not point out the flaws and limitations of their proposed ideas.

Q5: How would you prove the existence of life on Mars?

Applicant: I would want to know what is meant by 'life'- whether it means something Earth-like, or a more general definition. Then I would want either direct or indirect evidence. Direct evidence would be observing life itself, and the indirect would be observing some marker for this life based on how it was defined. Thus, I'll <u>start by thinking about how I would define life and then think about potential markers for it.</u>

This is a practical question that aims to set out what the hypotheses would be for future experiments. It is not about describing one precise experiment, but how you would design a series of experiments. With that in mind, it's important to ensure that suggested evidence is precisely defined, observable and measurable or quantifiable and repeatable because these features open the door to a great variety of experiment types. Thus, the response, "I'd like to see something that's alive" isn't quite detailed enough. You can suggest something which is currently impossible, such as wanting to observe a specimen drilled from one kilometre down on Mars, but should include some practical ideas as well.

One approach would be to define life as an <u>ability to create chemical disequilibria</u>. Through respiration and other basic life functions, organisms shuffle electrons and molecules and create small disequilibria that are later used to power life functions (consider photosynthesis and the shuffling of electrons from donors to acceptors using sunlight to power the process). The surface and atmosphere could be studied for disequilibria, starting with those associated with life on Earth.

There are many other possible approaches, but the general idea is to define the question more specifically and then suggest <u>possible evidence</u> which could be found in a range of experiments. You should suggest multiple experiments as it is necessary to have a sizeable data-pool before reaching a conclusion on such a broad question.

Q6: Why don't we have more than two eyes? Why do we only have one mouth?

This is a question that involves disentangling ultimate and proximate causes. When answering this question, it is important to show that you can approach a question from a variety of perspectives, including both <u>Proximate Causes</u> about <u>how the mechanism</u> influences the observed condition, but also <u>Ultimate Causes</u> about <u>why</u> this may be and what <u>function</u> this serves- particularly from an adaptive standpoint.

For a complete answer to this question, both types of cause are important. Take a moment to consider this from a few perspectives:

- A mechanistic approach through which eyes and mouths work.
- An evolutional approach by considering adaptation and fitness/survival and its impact on biological designs.
- An anthropological approach by considering evolutionary history and how our ancient ancestors influence the bodies we have today.

How many eyes and mouths we have is a matter of trade-offs: one eye provides an image of the surroundings, but <u>depth perception is only possible with two or more</u>. The slightly different angle from each eye allows us to determine how far away each object is. A very close object will project a very different image in each eye, while distant objects will look the same. The brain is then able to compare the differences in the images in order to estimate distances.

Having an extra eye and being able to integrate the two images is metabolically expensive energetically as a significant amount of neural processing is required. The gains from coordination in capturing prey and escaping predators offsets these costs, allowing for the second eye. A third eye could be helpful as it would allow vision ahead and behind simultaneously. However, each additional eye would be increasingly costly as its image would need to be integrated with the other eyes. Thus, the gains from escaping predators or spotting prey wouldn't be offset.

However, you might also point out that given rampant obesity and other signs that humans have great amounts of spare energy, it would now make sense to have an extra number of eyes. Similarly, for common prey, the metabolic costs of an additional eye could be offset by increased survival.

A mouth is the point of access to the digestive system and only one is required to ingest nutrients. Thus, having more mouths would mean an increase to the rate at which we could ingest food. However, a larger mouth could achieve similar results, so the energetic costs of growing a second fully-functioning mouth are not supported. In addition, introducing another mouth would increase the <u>risk of infections</u>.

There is another dimension to this question than the <u>how</u> and <u>why</u>- the <u>was</u>. Humans can't just grow another mouth or gazelles another eye because our ancestors did not have these. We have no genes to produce this extremely complex and divergent phenotype. It does not matter whether the prey would benefit from the third eye or not- they just can't grow one instantly because the path to that design is too difficult to attain from the present two eye setup.

In general, it is not easy to make such drastic physical changes (even over long periods of time). For example, consider the opposite case: if our ancestors had evolved a three-eye-system. The species would be more likely to become extinct rather than transform to a two-eye system.

A <u>poor applicant</u> would miss the point of this question- it is not to delve deeply into the workings of 3D vision and the digestive system, or even into trade-offs in an adaptation that lead to limits on designs. The point is to show that <u>there are many perspectives which must be integrated</u> to fully consider a question as complex as this.

Q7: Can you liken DNA to sheet music?

A question like this is a great chance to demonstrate your lateral thinking skills. In any comparison question, <u>you should directly relate one thing to the other</u>. For example:

- DNA consists of different patterns of amino acids; sheet music consists of different patterns of 12 notes.
- DNA describes the order in which mRNA should be produced; sheet music describes the order in which the music should be played.
- DNA and sheet music can both contain instructions on how and when to repeat sections.
- Mistakes in reading DNA can result in harmful mutations – mistakes in reading sheet music can result in a ruined melody/chord.
- Mistakes in reading DNA can sometimes be beneficial and lead to useful mutations; mistakes in reading sheet music can also rarely make the piece better than it was originally written.

Q8: Do you have a favourite protein?

This question allows you to demonstrate your enthusiasm for the subject. <u>All answers are perfectly acceptable</u> as long as you can justify them. Do not waste a question like this on an answer which doesn't show specific biological knowledge.

For example, you might like <u>haemoglobin</u> because it is very important as it facilitates oxygen transfer, or because there are many interesting diseases associated with it, e.g. Sick Cell, Thalassaemia. Alternatively, you might like insulin because of its importance in blood glucose homeostasis or its relationship with diabetes.

Q9: Why should we care about the Hayflick Limit?

Firstly, if you do not know what the Hayflick Limit is, ASK! It is impossible to answer this question if you do not know this technical definition. The Hayflick Limit is the theoretical limit to the number of times a normal human cell can divide. A good approach to this question would be to start by <u>defining the Hayflick Limit</u> and suggesting proximate reasons for its existence e.g. shortening telomeres with each cell division until they reach a critical length. Then, if you have any suggestions for ultimate reasons, discuss those, e.g. older DNA is more mutated, so older cells are less healthy and less related to the original than younger cells. If you have time, you could show an interest in biological issues by discussing some implications you may know about deriving from this topic, referencing articles or other media e.g. documentaries or the highly recommended TED talks available online.

Examples of things that are relevant would be the stability of clones derived from mature DNA, the possibility of immortality with finite cell rejuvenation, or problems with cancer cells that exceed the Hayflick Limit. You aren't expected to have any significant knowledge of these – the interviewers would guide you throughout the process.

Q10: Why is the liver on the right side of the body?

This is another classic question about <u>disentangling ultimate and proximate causes</u>, mechanisms and functions. The actual answer doesn't matter - only that you can show that you are able to approach biological questions from different perspectives. You could take a proximate mechanism approach and argue that there is a reason the liver can only work in that position - perhaps it needs to be in a specific orientation to allow the other organs to fit into the human body in this right-hand configuration.

From an ultimate perspective, you could argue there is an evolutionary advantage to this configuration. Maybe it is advantageous to have the vital liver on the opposite side of the body to the equally vital heart in case of severe injury to one side. You could take an evolutionary history approach- that there is no advantage to having the liver on the right, but some ancient ancestor had a right-left asymmetry with right-hand organs which became the liver. The important part of this answer is to show you are not locked into one perspective, but that you can see the variety of biological factors which may be at work.

The last example to drive this point home would be the question, *"Why are flowers usually never green?"* You could argue this from a proximate perspective- that flowers aren't photosynthetically active and thus don't have green chlorophyll. Alternatively, you could approach it from an ultimate perspective- flowers are meant to be attractive to pollinators and thus need to stand out from the foliage. Therefore, their functionality would be diminished if they were green.

Q11: Why do humans have two ears?

This type of question is often asked because all good candidates should be able to arrive at the correct answer (even if they haven't heard of it before). Therefore, it is useful to <u>talk through your thought process</u>, which will also allow the interviewer to guide you if necessary. A good place to start is to recognise that there must be a distinct evolutionary advantage of having two ears, so it must allow for functions that are not possible to the same extent with only one ear.

Having two ears allows you to <u>compare differences in stimuli</u>. How could comparing the sound you hear in each ear be useful? The properties of this sound would include amplitude, frequency, and timing – why would these differ between the ears?

If sound is coming from one side of the head then it would reach one ear before the other, so the timing of the sound would differ between the ears. Similarly, the amplitude would also differ between the ears if the source was not equidistant from them. Finally, if a moving sound source is closer to one ear than the other, then its frequency will differ between the ears (an extrapolation of the Doppler Effect).

Therefore, a comparison of the timing, amplitude, and frequency of sounds in each ear provides the brain with enough information to allow sound localisation, which is a powerful evolutionary advantage.

Q12: Can you explain how the brain works in a single word?

The challenge of this question is that the brain is such a complex organ that no single word could ever summarise how it works. It is important to make it explicit to the interviewer that you recognise this. Secondly, you need to recognise that the question is about 'how' the brain works, so the best answers will talk about a process and not simply the architecture that allows it to work. For example, answering 'plasticity' would be more appropriate than answering 'synapses' or 'circuits. Whatever word you choose, the crucial thing is that you try to reasonably justify your answer.

A good student who chose 'plasticity' might then say: "this is because plasticity at the synaptic level encompasses processes like long-term potentiation and long-term depression. These are crucial in how the neural circuits that underlie brain function develop. Thus, they're ultimately responsible for modulating how one neuron responds to another neuron's firing and so how the circuits as a whole function. The crucial role of plasticity has been demonstrated in numerous brain functions; including learning, memory, emotions, sensation and the recovery from injury".

Q13: Is cancer inevitable?

This question is purposefully vague, so it is up to you to <u>specify what you think they are asking</u>. It also gives you scope to pick an angle for your answer through which you can best demonstrate your knowledge. You could take a <u>'nature vs. nurture'</u> approach, discussing how there is a genetic component to cancer that predisposes to or protects vs. cancer.

You should make it clear that it is the predisposition to cancer that could be considered inevitable, not cancer itself. <u>Mention any examples</u> you may know of, such as the association of mutation in the BRCA1 gene with breast cancer.

In general, cancer is a disease of ageing and <u>the risk of most cancers increases with age</u>. Thus, one could argue that if most people lived long enough, they would eventually get some type of cancer. Alternatively, you could argue that whilst getting cancer is inevitable at the moment (like getting an infection), medical advances may change this in the future. The important thing is to <u>define the question so that you are able to tackle it</u> rather than giving a one-word response.

Q14: Why do second messenger systems exist?

You may have learned about this topic in A-levels but may not have thought about why it is the way it is. The interviewer would give you a quick explanation of 2nd messengers if you hadn't heard of them before. Again, they are interested in how you deduce your answers logically and using first principles.

It is useful to think about why secondary messenger systems would have evolved and what <u>alternative systems</u> are conceivable. One such alternative is signalling chemicals that pass into the target cells and interact directly with effector proteins (such as steroid signalling). What advantages are conveyed by having an extra step in the signalling cascade?

This is best thought about in the context of an example, such as the cyclic adenosine monophosphate (cAMP) system and gives you an opportunity to display what you know about these systems. Having a system that requires binding of a primary messenger (e.g. acetylcholine) to a cell surface receptor (e.g. G-protein coupled receptors) allows for signals to be determined by receptor density to a certain extent. Similarly, a variety of <u>intracellular signalling</u> can affect the levels of a secondary messenger, allowing even finer control of the ultimate intracellular signal and response.

Perhaps most importantly, second messengers help to amplify the cellular response. For example, a single molecule of Acetylcholine (primary messenger) can result in millions of downstream 2nd messengers. This setup <u>allows cells to react to small stimuli very rapidly</u>.

Q15: Over the past century, which medical advancement would you judge to be the most significant?

There is no single right answer for this question- you just need to be able to justify your response. It is a good idea to pick something you may have read a little about so that you can <u>add detail to support your answer</u>. Some good options include antibiotics, population-scale vaccines (smallpox, polio and MMR are good examples), evidence-based analysis (placebo-controlled, blinded, randomised-controlled trials; meta-analysis), advances in blood typing/banking/infusion.

For example, "I think that the development of a huge array of antibiotics since the discovery of penicillin is perhaps the most important medical advance in the last 100 years. This is because bacterial infections are very common and affect most of us at some point in our lives. Before antibiotics, even very small infections could be life threatening. The discovery of antibiotics represented a paradigm shift in medicine whereby a huge number of very harmful infectious diseases (such as tuberculosis, diphtheria, typhoid) became treatable. Furthermore, antibiotics made surgery a lot safer, by reducing the risks of post-operative infection.

Your answer to this question may <u>determine the future line of questioning</u> for the remainder of the interview so choose carefully! For example, this particular response may lead to a discussion of how antibiotic resistance develops or why multi-drug resistant bacteria are a problem.

Q16: How would you plot a graph of drug concentration in the blood against time, for a drug partially removed by the kidneys prior to each subsequent dose?

You haven't been given enough information to allow you to draw the graph accurately e.g. the rate of absorption, the rate of elimination, and the time between each dose. However, you can still <u>draw the general shape</u> - as the drug is absorbed from the gut, the concentration of drug in the blood (called plasma drug concentration, or C) will rapidly increase.

When the majority of the drug has been absorbed, the <u>rate of drug elimination will exceed the rate of absorption</u>. Thus, there will be a turning point where C starts to decrease. C will continue to drop until the next dose.

Since the dose isn't fully eliminated, the lowest value of C will still be greater than zero. It will then again rapidly increase because the new dose is being absorbed.

Therefore, over several successive doses, C will become progressively greater to eventually give a graph shaped like below:

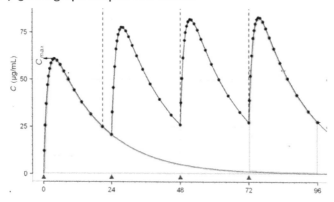

Q17: What does the nocebo effect tell us about how patients respond to treatment?

A good place to start with answering this question is to make it clear that you understand the difference between the 'nocebo effect' and negative iatrogenic side-effects produced by treatments. The key difference is that there is no physiological reason for the side-effects with the nocebo effect. You can then compare this to the well known 'placebo effect', where positive effects are experienced in response to 'drugs' (often completely inert sugar pills), despite there being no physiological explanation for this.

It is thought that the placebo effect is due to the patient's expectation of positive effects from the drug. Therefore, you could suggest that in nocebo, it is likely that some expectation of negative side effects could precipitate the perception of these negative side effects. Both these effects show that there is a psychological aspect to how patients respond to their treatments. This is very important when doctors consider how to manage patient expectations about how a treatment will affect them. It introduces an interesting ethical dilemma about keeping patients fully informed about the potential negative side effects of a treatment — it is important to let patients know the risks. However, doing this could cause them to experience negative side effects due to the 'nocebo effect'.

Q18: Why do humans rely on negative feedback?

You will know of examples of negative feedback from A-level Biology, such as homeostatic mechanisms like temperature control and the maintenance of steady blood glucose levels using insulin and glucagon. Although it's good to start by describing the role of negative feedback in these processes, it is crucial that you go on to discuss why homeostasis is necessary in the first place.

At the system level, you can discuss how using negative feedback to keep such parameters within a small range allows for larger physiological responses to relatively small changes in the environment. At the cellular level, the internal environment must be tightly regulated by negative feedback to allow enzymes to function efficiently e.g. temperature and pH.

A poor candidate would just list examples of negative feedback rather than discussing its significance.

Q19: What happens when the adrenal glands become hyperactive?

Your ability to answer this question will depend on if you know what hormones are produced by the adrenals and what their function is. Again, the interviewer will prompt you if you get stuck. The adrenals produce catecholamines such as adrenaline and noradrenaline as well as other steroid hormones like cortisol and aldosterone. Therefore, a 'hyperactive' adrenal gland would produce excess amounts of these hormones.

Catecholamines increase the heart rate and cause peripheral vasoconstriction. So increased catecholamine production from a hyperactive adrenal gland would lead to all of these features. You could also think about what would cause the adrenals to be 'hyperactive' e.g. an adrenal tumour or increased stimulation from the nerves innervating the adrenal gland.

Similarly, if you were aware of the effects of increased steroid hormones, then you should describe what actions they have and what would happen if there were increased production of them.

NB: This is an interesting area of clinical medicine and if you're interested in endocrinology – you are advised to do some background reading on *Cushing's Syndrome* and *Conn's Syndrome*.

Q20: What diseases do you think we should screen for?

This ethical question gives you an opportunity to demonstrate an understanding of resource allocation and knowledge of any screening programmes that you are aware of. You can discuss how it is important that the resources are used to achieve the most benefit for the most people (utilitarian argument). This is often measured using quality adjusted life-years (QUALYs) by the National Institute of Health and Care Excellence (NICE). They perform these calculations in order to decide if screening is appropriate. So for screening to be appropriate and cost-effective:

- The disease must be an important health problem
- The disease should be treatable
- There should be a simple screening test for the disease
- The test should have low false positive and false negative rates
- The test should be cost-effective

You could then offer your opinion on which diseases would satisfy these criteria. For completeness, current screening programmes include:

- Pap smears vs. Cervical Cancer
- Mammograms vs. Breast cancer
- Faecal Occult blood test vs. Colorectal cancer
- Foetal blood tests for Down's Syndrome

Q21: Why do you want to be a doctor?

What this question is exploring: This question is investigating your motivation behind medicine. It is extremely likely to come up so is definitely worth thinking about. Why do you actually want to become a doctor? What is it about the profession that appeals to you? Why do you want to go into medicine and not other healthcare professions e.g. nursing, pharmacy, occupational therapy?

Tips for a good answer:

- *Explain that your motivation for medicine has grown over many experiences.* This is a good way to involve work experience and extra-curricular work e.g. extra reading and attending lectures.

- *Make it personal to you* - pretty much all candidates will say something along the lines of being interested in the sciences and wanting to do something with people. Try and think of things that will make you stand out e.g. doing a research project about a new drug in your spare time and seeing the day-to-day life of a consultant during work experience.

- Show that you know what being a doctor involves - talk about the responsibilities of doctors This will also show you know the differences between doctors and other healthcare professionals e.g. nurses often take blood and perform ECGs but it is a doctor's role to interpret them and choose a plan of management from there.
  - Show that you understand medicine is a life-long degree and you are able to take this on

- Give examples about specific aspects of medicine which appeal to you

Model answer:

I want to be a doctor as I enjoy scientific academia which stimulates my learning, as well as the social aspect of engaging with patients in a clinical setting. Science has always interested me. Over the last few years, my interest in human biology has developed into a passion after attending lectures by the Royal Society on topics ranging from pain relief to cataracts. I have also gained a detailed insight into the duties and responsibilities of a doctor through many work experience placements, including shadowing a consultant in a paediatric ICU last summer. Seeing the process of reaching a diagnosis and deciding on courses of treatment showed me how intellectually stimulating this career is and specifically appeals to me as I relish problem-solving and being academically challenged (as shown by achieving a gold award in a national chemistry Olympiad). Whilst volunteering at a local hospice I also appreciated the emotional side of medicine, with doctors having to have difficult conversations with relatives. I feel like I would be able to take on the emotional challenges of being a doctor and this would enable me to make a difference to patients' lives on a daily basis.

Avoid:

- Not giving evidence about why you want to be a doctor
- Making sweeping statements e.g. doctors have to deal with life-or-death decisions every day
- Talking about how prestigious the job is/money
- Generic or unrealistic answers e.g. I had an operation as a child and from then knew I wanted to be a doctor

Q22: Take a look at this skull. What can you learn about it?

What this question is exploring: The interviewers will present you with a foreign object. You may have some idea about what it is, but they want to see you think out loud and work on the spot.

Tips for a good answer:

- Describe exactly what you see in front of you
  - E.g. what colour is it? How big is it? What animal is it likely to come from? What features can you recognise on the skull? Are there any injuries/deformities?
- Talk through your answer
  - The examiners want to see how you think so make sure you are talking out loud for every part of your answer, even if it is extremely obvious!
- If you don't know - still say something
  - If they have given you something you don't know anything about, voice an opinion and they will help you if you get stuck. They want to keep you going until you get to the 'end' of the question
- Don't rush- take your time and properly examine the object

Model answer: This is a skull of an animal. It is about 15x20x20cm in shape and is a pale white colour. The shape is relatively elliptical, with a relatively narrow face and extended length from back to front. It has large recesses for its eyes, which might mean it uses good vision for catching prey. I think it probably comes from a

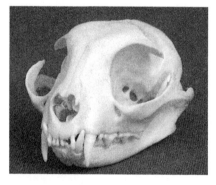

small mammal of the feline family e.g. a cat. I am thinking this due to its size, shape (long back to front) and its teeth. I am looking at the teeth now and this animal seems to be a carnivore due to its big incisors. I can also identify two large orbital recesses which is where the eyes would be.

I think it is too small to be the skull of a big cat and so I am more likely to think of it as being from a domesticated cat. There are no obvious deformities to the skull, and it looks healthy.

Avoid:

- Not describing it fully and just stating that it is a skull
- Going off on a tangent about something unrelated e.g. the function of every type of tooth
- Not thinking aloud and explaining every aspect to the interviewer.

Q23: Tell me the number of petrol stations in Europe.

What this question is exploring: This is a question asking you about your estimation/maths skills. They will present you with a strange question which might seem random at first but the thinking behind this is fairly logical. Good maths skills and critical thinking are vital to Oxbridge medicine.

Tips for a good answer:

- Be methodical - try and think of how many petrol stations are in a town/city. Then how many towns/cities/service stations there might be in a country. Then what the average size of a country is in Europe. Then how many countries there are in Europe.
- Try and estimate values - don't be too specific or multiplication will get very tricky
- Think out loud - if you just come up with a random value the interviewers will not be impressed no matter how close this is - they want to see your thought process and how you come to the answer.

Model answer: I am going to use the UK an as example of a European country. Let me first think of how many petrol stations there are in an average town/city. I think there may be roughly 0.5 in a town and 10 in a city. We also have to think of how many there will be in services along motorways (I estimate there will be around 1000 service stations along motorways in the UK). I think, in European countries (which are well developed), there will be around 15 cities, 15,000 towns and 5000 villages. This would mean, in an average country there would be $(10*15) + (0.5*15,000) + 1000$. This means in the UK there would be roughly 9000 petrol stations. I think the UK is representative of a higher-than-average country in terms of population, so will multiply this by 0.5 to give around 4500 in an average country. There are around 40 countries in Europe so my final answer would be $4500*40 =$ roughly 200,000.

Avoid:

- Not explaining - it doesn't matter if you get it completely wrong - they just want to see your logic
- Being too precise - don't forget you have a limited time to answer
- Thinking too 'out of the box' - usually these questions are actually quite straightforward and just require simple maths

Q24: What makes a cheetah so fast?

What this question is exploring: This question is asking about your knowledge of anatomy and physiology. This is a good opportunity to show tutors your analytical skills integrated into science whilst exploring something you may not have learnt about before.

Tips for a good answer:

- Structure your answer
  - If you are going to talk about different components working together, make sure you group them together (e.g. talking first about cardiovascular changes, then respiratory, then musculoskeletal)
- Try and be accurate with your science
  - Instead of saying 'the cheetah's back can bend to extreme amounts' use proper scientific terms (the spine can withstand high levels of flexion and extension) to show the interviewers you know what you are talking about
- Ask the interviewers for prompts
  - This is a fairly scientific question so if you don't know the answer straight away, don't panic! Ask your tutor for prompts to help you get to the right answer and try and give an answer that will make them lead you down the right path e.g. the animal has a similar skeleton and muscle mass to other feline relatives so it must have special adaptations in how it moves
- Explain why structural changes relate to function

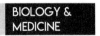

Model answer: The cheetah can accelerate from 0-60mph at the same rate as a Ferrari. Unlike other feline relatives, it has special adaptations to its anatomy and physiology in order to achieve this. In terms of differences in anatomy, we can start by looking at the cardiovascular system. Firstly, the cheetah has an enlarged heart and large arteries which allow high levels of blood to perfuse respiring muscles around the body and allows for a rapid rate of gas exchange. Moreover, in the respiratory system, the cat has enlarged lungs to allow for a large volume of oxygen to be taken in with every breath, ensuring enough oxygen is delivered to tissues. The cheetah's most unique feature; however, is a spine which allows for extreme flexion and extension whilst running, allowing for a greater reach of its front and hind legs, allowing the cat to cover a greater distance per stride. Finally, its legs also display special characteristics; in these cats, the tibia and fibula are fused, allowing for higher levels of stability at speed. The paw pads of the cheetah are also hard and less rounded than other wild cats, allowing for increased traction.

Avoid:
- Talking about adaptations and not explaining *how* they allow a cheetah to run at top speeds
- Hesitate if you don't know the answer - the tutors will guide you, it is best to give a logical guess that it needs to have an extremely efficient cardiovascular system and changes to its musculoskeletal system
- Comparing a cheetah to humans - a wild cat is obviously going to run faster than us, comparing it to its feline counterparts highlights the specialist adaptations and why the cheetah is so unique

Q25: What makes a horse's leg so well-suited to running?

What this question is exploring: This questions the student's knowledge of anatomy. This is a good opportunity to show tutors your analytical skills integrated into science whilst exploring something you may not have learnt about before.

Tips for a good answer:

- Talk through anatomy in a structured way
  - o Start with the bones, then muscle, then hooves etc. This shows the interviewers you are thinking in a methodical way.
- Use correct anatomical terms
  - o Instead of saying bend and straighten the leg, use flex and extend instead.
- Ask the interviewers for prompts
  - o This is a fairly scientific question so if you don't know the answer straight away, don't panic! Start off with what you know about the leg of a mammal, then think about how the anatomy may be adapted to running. Even if the answer is wrong, it shows that you are thinking along the right lines and are giving reasonable suggestions. This should make the interviewer help you to think of the correct adaptations.
- Extra credit - why is it important for horses to be quick? (To outrun predators etc)

Model answer: The horse's leg is adapted to running as it needs to reach high speeds in order to avoid predators. The long bones pivot on pulley-like joints, allowing large strides to be taken by the animal. Moreover, the horse does not have a collarbone, meaning that the front legs are attached to the axial skeleton by a plethora of muscles and ligaments, allowing for freedom of movement of these legs. Furthermore, the horse does not have a large amount of muscle in its distal leg, most of the muscle mass is concentrated above the knee. This allows stride rate to be increased during running, as there is less mass for the knee to flex and extend. Finally, the horse walks permanently on the tips of its toes, allowing for full extension of the limbs in running. This enables it to cover a larger distance per stride. The hooves of the horse also provide support, traction and shock absorption. This allows the horse to run at speed for long distances whilst minimising the risk of injury.

Avoid:

- Talking about adaptations and not explaining *how* they allow horses to run
- Randomly listing everything you know about the leg
  - If you don't boil your answer down to what is relevant to the question, the examiners will question whether you are able to academically analyse a simple question and formulate a relevant answer
- Comparing the horse's leg to a human's - this has nothing to do with the question. The question is asking how the leg is adapted, rather than a comparison.

Q26: Tell me about your favourite animal.

What this question is exploring: This may seem simple on the surface, but this is more of a conversation starter than a question itself. In medicine/veterinary interviews these types of questions give the interviewers a starting point to delve deeper into why things are the way they are. E.g. the conversation may start with 'what is your favourite animal?' but will probably go down the route of 'why does this animal have this adaptation?' and 'why is this important for its survival' or 'how does this adaptation work?'

Tips for a good answer:

- Know a bit about your choice
  - This is crucial when the interviewers ask follow-up questions. If you used the example of a bat and mentioned their use of sonar for being able to detect objects in the dark, it is crucial you know how this works.
- Think in a scientific way
  - The interviewers are likely to delve deep into the science behind what makes the animal unique. Usually, adaptations come about because they provide some sort of evolutionary advantage e.g. aye-aye's have extremely long fingers so they are able to dig bugs out of tree trunks. If you do not know why an adaptation exists, try and think if this allows the animal to avoid predators/catch prey/find a mate.

- Keep going!
  - o With these types of questions examiners will usually dig quite deep, but it's ok to not know everything and feel free to ask the interviewers for some guidance along the way.

Model answer:

- 'My favourite animal probably has to be the hammerhead shark. It is a unique predator which has a relatively flat head and eyes which are found on the distal protrusions of its head. I love it because its shape is so distinctive and is known as an extremely fierce predator in the animal kingdom'
- 'Great! What an interesting animal. Why do you think a flat head would give the animal an advantage in feeding or survival?'
- 'It's head shape is designed specifically to be able to pin down animals. For example, when hunting, the shark can pin stingrays down with its flat head. The fact that its eyes are on the ends of these two prominences means that it has a really wide field of vision, this is also probably good to spot prey.'
- 'Brilliant- let's now think about how the head of this animal is formed. When the shark is an embryo, how does the body know to form this shape?'
- 'I'm not really sure but it might have something to do with gene expression and signalling? So if molecular signals move away from a place that is controlling growth and they can't be picked up anymore, growth might stop?'
- etc...

Avoid:

- Choosing an animal you know nothing about because you think it will impress them
  - o Once they start digging around it will be obvious that you don't know your stuff
- Choosing a pet
  - o Although you may love your dog/cat/hamster very dearly, these animals usually do not have a large amount of interesting science to talk about and might bore the interviewers

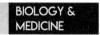
Q27: Why is an elephant's foot structured as it is?

What this question is exploring: This question is asking about your knowledge of anatomy and physiology. Although there are some details to this answer which you may not know about, it is a good opportunity to show tutors your analytical skills and your ability to think logically when presented with an odd question. Rather than knowing the specifics about how the elephant's foot is special, this is an opportunity to test your scientific thinking and explore *why* the foot has these adaptations.

Tips for a good answer:

- Talk through anatomy in a structured way
    - Start with the general structure, then bones, then muscle etc. This shows the interviewers you are thinking in a methodical way.
- Use correct anatomical terms
    - E.g. Instead of saying bend and straighten the leg, use flex and extend instead.
- Explain **why** in addition to **how**
    - Although it is good to explain how the elephant's foot has special adaptation, you need to explain why the adaptations actually occur - e.g. the padding allows for the protection of and important sensitive structures such as blood vessels and nerves *rather than* there is padding on the elephant's foot.
- Link to clinical problems if you can

Model answer: Elephants can weigh up to 6,000 kg. The elephant's foot is designed in a way to minimise damage which would occur to the immense pressure put on it by carrying an enormous amount of weight. Firstly, the circumference of the foot is extremely large compared to other animals. This allows large amounts of pressure generated by the elephant's weight to be spread over a large area, imperative for the bones to be able to withstand the huge force generated by the animal's weight. Furthermore, the presence of distal cushions of adipose tissue in the elephant's foot allow for structures such as tendons and ligaments to be protected from the large weight of the elephant's body. It is important for these structures not to be compressed as this can lead to pathologies such as tendonitis and movement difficulties.

Avoid:
- Not explaining *why* the foot has these special adaptations
  - Just stating that it has a large surface area to support a big weight is not enough detail. You must think more critically e.g. the elephant needs to spread its weight out over a large surface area as it often comes into contact with mud and soft ground (when drinking) and so needs to be able to navigate this terrain without getting stuck.
- Listing facts quickly
  - This does not show the interviewer that you are considering the question in depth and being critical of the question. It is important to show that you are being pushed out of your comfort zone as this is what the interviews aim to do.

Q28: Describe the function of an electron microscope.

What this question is exploring: This is a basic science question. It is aiming to understand something you should have covered at A level and they are likely to show you example images to discuss later.

Tips for a good answer:

- Know your stuff
  - Before Oxbridge interviews, it is a good idea to look at what you have been covering in A level science and some common topics which may come up e.g. haemoglobin dissociation curve, Kreb's cycle, microscopy, DNA replication and transgene editing.
- Try to give examples
  - What have you seen in your biology lessons associated with light microscopy? You could talk about specific organelles in a cell which are only visible by this method e.g. cristae of mitochondria
- Compare it with light microscopy for bonus points
  - Understanding different methods of microscopy will come across very well to the interviewers and sometimes it is even easier explaining something when you can compare and contrast.
- Talk about the different types
  - Scanning vs transmission
- Draw a diagram!

Model answer:

Electron microscopes utilise the same main concepts that a light microscope uses. In light microscopy, you need a light source, a specimen, and a lens to magnify the image. Electron microscopy uses the same concepts, but with slightly different materials: electrons as the light source (these allow for a high resolution to be obtained), a specimen (frozen) and

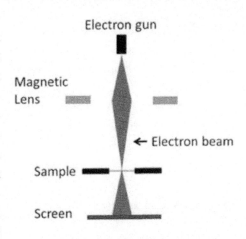

electromagnets replacing the lens (these focus the electron beams). First, a beam of electrons is fired through the sample. The electromagnets speed this beam up, causing the beam to act in a similar way to light waves. Another magnet then focuses the beam and produces the magnified image. There are two main types of electron microscopy: transmission (TEM) and scanning (SEM). TEM is used to investigate slices of biological specimens whilst SEM is used to examine the surface structure, due to a large depth of field. These are both vital in biomedical science, as they allow high-resolution images of extremely small biological components to be seen e.g. the internal structure of mitochondria.

Avoid:

- Overcomplicating your answer
  - This is a relatively straightforward question, give a concise and accurate answer so the interviewers can ask you more in-depth questions to stretch your thinking
- Not explaining it fully
  - Act as though the interviewers know nothing about microscopy. This will make sure that you will give a full answer which does not miss anything key out!

Q29: How do dolphins regulate their body temperature?

What this question is exploring: This is a simple question testing your knowledge of homeostasis and how animals use adaptations to survive in warmer or cooler temperatures. Even though you may not know exactly how it works in dolphins, use your knowledge of homeostasis in mammals. It is important to understand the neural pathways by which this happens as they are likely to ask follow up questions as: *'How does a dolphin know if it is in hot or cold water?'* or *'how does the dolphin know when to stop increasing or decreasing its body temperature?'*

Tips for a good answer:

- Structure your answer
  - It is good to talk about different components to the answer separately. First, mention homeostasis and how an internal body temperature is maintained regardless of water temperature. Then talk about specialist adaptations dolphins have to aid temperature control.
- Draw diagrams
  - If you are able to, this will make explaining homeostasis easier and will show that you are very confident in both speaking about this topic and presenting your ideas in a pictorial way (very important for science!)
- Mention adaptations at the end
  - If you have time, talk about how these animals have a small surface area to volume ratio (SA:V), have lots of blubber to protect them from the cold and also undergo seasonal migration to warmer waters.
- Be ready for follow up questions on temperature sensing and how blood flow is controlled within the body!

Model answer:

Like other mammals, dolphins are warm-blooded, and so need to maintain a constant internal temperature despite their surroundings. This process is known as *homeostasis*. The process can be seen in this diagram below, with the main thermoregulatory

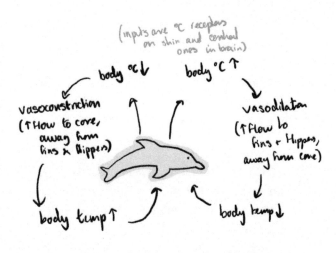

(inputs are °C receptors on skin and central ones in brain)

body °C ↓   body °C ↑

vasoconstriction
(↑ flow to core, away from fins & flippers)

vasodilation
(↑ flow to fins + flippers, away from core)

body temp ↑   body temp ↓

mechanism being the redirection of blood flow within the mammal (explain as drawing diagram). Moreover, dolphins have behavioural and physiological adaptations that allow the maintenance of a constant internal temperature. Firstly, they are highly migratory, allowing them to dodge extreme external conditions. Dolphins also have many physical adaptations. Firstly, they have a small SA:V, allowing them the conserve body heat more efficiently. Dolphins also have a layer of blubber which helps with insulation. They also have a low exhalation rate compared to other mammals, helping them to keep in warm air and further conserve body heat.

Avoid: talking about human adaptations - dolphins don't have hair and shiver/sweat!

Q30: How do reflexes in the leg work? How would this be affected if the spinal cord were damaged at the level of the neck?

What this question is exploring: This is a basic reflex arc question. Know your science.

The second part is a bit trickier and is trying to make you think outside the box/think critically about a question you have probably not considered before.

Tips for a good answer:

- Define what a reflex is
- Tackle the question in two separate parts
    - Describe a reflex arc and show you understand how it works
    - Talk about what would happen in the leg
- Give examples of reflexes
    - Ankle jerk, knee jerk etc.
- Draw a diagram
    - Reflex arcs can be simplified by drawing a diagram. There will usually be a whiteboard and pens in the room to do this with, but a pencil and paper will suffice! This will show that you are very confident in both speaking about this topic and presenting your ideas in a pictorial way (very important for science!)

Model answer:

Reflexes are extremely important in the human body; they are involuntary movements arising from a stimulus and do not require neural pathways to or from the brain. Examples of these include the knee jerk reflex (patellar tendon) and the ankle jerk reflex. As seen in the diagram to the right, sensory (afferent) neurons carry nerve impulses from stimuli towards the central nervous system, whilst

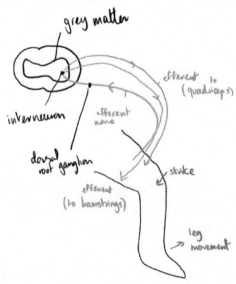

motor (efferent) neurons are motor neurons that carry neural impulses away from the CNS towards effector muscles. If the sensory neurons are stimulated, a reflex occurs. This depends on the site of stimulation - if the patellar tendon is hit, the knee extends. On the other hand, if the Achilles tendon is hit, plantarflexion is achieved. If the spinal cord was damaged at a site distant to this reflex, e.g. the neck, then the reflex would still occur, as it only involves the spinal cord segment closest to the leg.

Diagram explanation: A tendon hammer strikes the patellar tendon. This causes sensory receptors in the muscle to be stretched, stimulating the afferent sensory neuron. This passes through the dorsal root ganglion and into the grey matter of the spinal cord, where it synapses with an interneuron. This then synapses straight onto motor nerves which pass down to the appropriate leg muscles. The arc ends with an extension of the knee.

Q31: How many molecules of gas are in here?

What this question is exploring: This question wants you to apply A-level chemistry to the everyday world. It wants to assess your critical thinking skills whilst consolidating basic knowledge. These attributes are vital when looking for a good candidate.

Tips for a good answer:

- Be methodical
    - How many moles of gas are there in $1m^3$? How big is the room? What other factors do we have to consider? (e.g. temp, pressure)
- Try and estimate values
    - Don't be too specific or multiplication will get very tricky
- Think out loud
    - If you just come up with a random value the interviewers will not be impressed no matter how close this is - they want to see your thought process and how you come to the answer.
- Ask for paper to write notes on if it helps you think

Model answer:

- Assuming normal temp + pressure
- x = volume of room (m^3)

$$pV = nRT$$

$p = 100,000 \, Pa$

$n = ?$

$T = (25 + 273) = 298k$

$V = x \, m^3$

$R = 8.31 \, Jk^{-1}mol^{-1}$

$$n = \frac{PV}{RT}$$

$$= \frac{100,000 \times x}{8.31 \times 298}$$

$$= 40.38 \, x \, (mol)$$

assuming this room = $300 \, m^3$

$$mol \approx 12,000 \text{ in this room}$$

(I used a random value for the volume of the room).
Mol=12,000 so there would be 6.02x10²³ * this value to figure out how many molecules there would be.

Alternate answer:
I mole of gas occupies 24 dm³ at room temperature and pressure, this is 0.024 m³. I estimate this room to be 10m x 10m x 30m, so 300m³. Thus, the estimated number of moles in the room is 300 ÷ 0.024. If I round 0.024 to 0.025 this is 1/40, so the answer is 300*40 ≈ 12,000 moles

Avoid:

• Not explaining - it doesn't matter if you get it completely wrong- they just want to see your logic
• Being too precise - don't forget you have a limited time to answer

Q32: How do fish respire? How is this different from mammals?

What this question is asking: This question is testing your knowledge of basic biological mechanisms in different animals. Having a sound knowledge of the process of human respiration will help answer the question, as it will push you to think about the differences between the anatomy and physiology between mammals and fish.

Tips for a good answer:

- Compare and contrast
  - Start with mammals first and then for every aspect of respiration you talk about, show how it is similar/different in fish. This will show the interviewers that you have a strategic way of thinking about an academic question.
- Think systematically
  - Start with a basic overview, then go more in detail about certain aspects of respiration e.g. start with the overall structure of the lungs and how gas exchange occurs, then compare how the gills in a fish differ structure by structure
- Use correct anatomical terms
- Explain why the different structures in fish exist - what would happen if fish had a nose/trachea/lungs like we do?

Model answer: In mammals, our respiratory apparatus consists of nasal passages, a trachea, bronchi, bronchioles and alveoli. We breathe in through our nose, air travels down these structures and ends at alveoli, which are sacs of air which are extremely well perfused, allowing gas exchange to take place. Fish, as well as mammals, need oxygen to survive; however, if they had the same respiratory apparatus that mammals have the lungs would fill with water and the fish would undergo a pleural effusion and eventually drown. They therefore have a different anatomy which still allows gas exchange to occur. Fish take in water through their mouth and then force it out through organs called gills. These usually sit laterally on either side of their neck and are synonymous to the lungs of mammals. Gills are made up of threadlike structures called filaments, supported by serrated branchial arches (calcium-based support structures). These filaments, like the alveoli, are highly vascularised, allowing for high amounts of gas exchange between the water and blood. Gasses diffuse between the water and blood by diffusion due to thin walls, as in the lungs. In many fish the capillary blood flow is in the opposite direction to the flow of water, allowing a countercurrent exchange to be created, further maximising the efficiency of gas exchange.

Avoid:
- Not comparing and contrasting
- Just saying fish have gills
  - What do they do? What do they replace in the mammal's respiratory system?

Q33: In a completely dissociated aqueous sulphuric acid solution at pH 2 - how many sulphate ions are there?

What this question is exploring: This is a basic chemistry question, assessing your knowledge of calculations and your ability to be put on the spot. Stay calm, go through the question methodically.

Tips for a good answer:

- Be methodical
  - How do we calculate [H+] from pH? How do we calculate [SO4^{2-}]? How do we calculate the number of ions?
- Think out loud
  - If you just come up with a random value the interviewers will not be impressed no matter how close this is - they want to see your thought process and how you come to the answer.

Model answer:

$$pH = -\log[H^+]$$

$$2 = -\log_{10}x$$

$$-2 = \log_{10}x$$

$$x = 10^{-2}$$

Thus the concentration of H$^+$ ions in the solution is 0.01 mol dm^{-3} so the concentration of SO42- ions is half that $0.005 \text{ mol dm}^{-3}$

In 0.5 L, there are 0.0025 mol of sulphate ions, so multiply this by Avogadro's constant to calculate the number of ions.

$$0.0025 \text{ mol} \times 6.02 \times 10^{23} \approx 1.5 \times 10^{21}$$

Avoid:

- Giving an answer and not explaining the steps you're going through
- Silly mistakes
  - E.g. forgetting you need to multiply by 2 as sulphuric acid has 2 protons in it/forgetting to multiply by Avogadro's constant at the end

Q34: What experiment would you design to test whether Female deer select their mates based on the size of their antlers if older deer have bigger antlers?

What this question is asking: This is a basic experimental design system. It is testing your basic experimental knowledge and is a relatively straightforward question. Make sure you don't forget the basics of how to design an experiment!

Tips for a good answer:

- Don't overcomplicate things
  - The best experiments are ones with clear aims and have a straight-forward method
- Define your variables
  - Control variables are extremely important - make sure you don't forget these

Model answer:

Independent variable:
- Antler mass (g)

Dependent variable:
- Mating success (as defined by number of calves produced over a 10-year period).

Control variables:
- Species of deer, body size

I would design an experiment whereby the size of antlers differs between males. I would measure antler size (g) and also measure overall weight of the animal to make sure I can control for body size. I would then record their success in terms of mating by measuring how many calves they produce. I would run this experiment over 10 years to involve a large portion of the mating period during their lifetime. I would only use adult males, who will be mating for the next 10 years of their lifetime. In this way, I would be able to see whether there is an associated between antler size (g) and breeding success (# calves).

Avoid:

- Not defining variables
- Not giving units for variables e.g. mass of antlers in grams

Q35: Male deer show-fight when competing for mates, rather than fighting to the death - is there an evolutionary point to this?

What this question is asking: This is assessing your knowledge of natural selection and evolution. Although it might seem like a bizarre question, the concept is simple: how is avoiding the death of mates evolutionary advantageous to the species?

Tips for a good answer:

- Define key terms
  - What is an evolutionary advantage? Why is this important?
- Think logically
  - Why would it be a good idea to conserve the life of males of the species?
- Use examples to illustrate your answer
  - If you ranked all the males in a group 1-100 from the 'best mate' to the 'worst mate', why would it be bad for #1 vs #2 to fight each other?

Model answer:

The process of evolution can be defined as the change in heritable characteristics of populations over many generations. This is necessary for the survival of a species, as it allows more individuals to survive in a certain environment. Selective mating is an essential aspect of evolution, as it allows only those who are 'biologically fit' to have offspring. In show-fighting, the idea is that the stronger male will win the fight and be able to mate and ensure that the next generation of deer will also be strong and fit. However, if males were to fight to the death, this would be detrimental to their species. Firstly, males mate many times, and so the numbers of the population would diminish by half rapidly. For example, if we start with 100 males and each male mates 4 times in each season, only 6 (.25) males would remain. This is obviously putting the species at a massive disadvantage as it quickly decreases the number of males which would be able to mate. Moreover, if we ranked all the males from 'best' to 'worst' in terms of desirable evolutionary characteristics, there is no guarantee #1 would not fight against #2 and so on. This means that, theoretically, you could actually get rid of some males which would make perfect mating partners.

Avoid:

- Not explaining your thoughts fully
  - Act as though the interviewers know nothing about evolution. This will make sure you will give a full answer that does not miss anything key out!
- Hesitate if you don't know the answer - the tutors will guide you, it is best to give a logical guess and explain your reasoning behind it than simply saying you don't know

Q36: How do you test which colours Rats and Octopuses can see?

What this question is exploring: This question wants you to apply some knowledge of colour vision from A-level biology and apply this in a research setting. It wants to assess your ability to formulate and describe a research study and is a good opportunity to display critical thinking and application of anatomy in an integrative context.

Tips for a good answer:

- It is not necessary to know the specific colours a rat or octopus can distinguish, or their specific neuroanatomy.
  - This question is all about your own interpretation – there is no specific correct answer! If you are making logical points from first principles, building on what you know of colour vision, the interviewers will help you if you are stuck on a specific fact.
- Talk through your answer through
  - The interviewers want to know your thought process and why you are coming up with the ideas you are voicing. This will also make it easier for you to develop your answer and build on what you have already said.
- Include some points about what would make a good research study
  - For example: How you could control your study? What are your variables? What hypothesis are you testing? This demonstrates knowledge about how important these factors are.
- Compare and contrast between the two parts of the question
  - Describe what you would do the same and differently for the rat and octopus, which will make for a well-structured answer.

Model answer: I would first investigate the photoreceptors in the retina, specifically the cone cells as these respond to light of different wavelengths to determine colour vision. I would use microscopy of the fovea and light wavelength studies to deduce the number, and type, of cone cells in the rat and octopus eye. This could be compared to human trichromatic vision.

I would then develop a research study, perhaps to train the rat to find the odd colour amongst a series of panels for a food reward. This would be more difficult with the octopus, where it may be necessary to place a coloured reward concealed by a background colour to test whether it can reach this. Control variables could be that the food reward is only distinguishable by sight; the environmental conditions remain the same each time; and the status of the animal is controlled each time (for example, hunger levels). It would be necessary to use multiple individuals of each species, to ensure it is a species-wide conclusion and not just for a specific animal. It would also be necessary to repeat the study many times for reliability, as the design provides an opportunity for the animals to demonstrate a 'positive result' by chance.

Avoid:

- Rushing in with everything you can think about colour vision
- Panicking that you don't know anything about animal colour vision – it is still possible to provide a critical, well-structured answer with no prior knowledge

Q37: What mutations could shorten or lengthen RNA or DNA?

What this question is exploring: This question is asking you to apply knowledge of mutations from A-level biology in a structured and logical way. There are many types of mutations and it is not necessary to specifically name them all, this is testing an ability to demonstrate understanding by categorising and explaining how this can come about. This is often taught in the context of how this mutated RNA or DNA codes for proteins through transcription and translation, so this question wants you to think about this from a different perspective.

Tips for a good answer:

- Try to use correct biological terms where you can
  - For example, point mutation, deletion, substitution
- Structure your answer in a logical way
  - This could be on scales, for example, smaller to larger scale mutations
- Demonstrate knowledge of the structure of DNA and RNA relevant to mutation
  - For example, genes and chromosomes
- Add some clinical relevance if possible

Model answer: Mutations can either be inherited or sporadic and affect the structure of the final protein product. The same categories of mutations can occur in RNA and DNA as these are both formed of the same nucleotide structure. These are all centred around the structure of a nucleotide sequence, with A, T, C and G bases which can be added or removed in a particular way to render the molecule longer or shorter. Not all mutations make DNA or RNA change length, for example, point mutations or substitutions. These mutations often occur during DNA replication if they are sporadic but can also be inherited. On a small scale, insertions and deletions describe where a base is added or removed from the sequence, so the molecule is one base length different. Duplications can also occur, where a small length of DNA is copied more than once. Repeat expansions occur when nucleotide repeats of short sequences are repeated more than they should be. On a larger scale, insertions and deletions can occur with many more base pairs, sometimes called a copy number variation. This can even be whole genes, sequences encoding for a protein product, being repeated or removed. On an even wider scale, chromosomal mutations can occur: chromosomes are a long DNA molecule containing genetic material, and loss of one or both copies of a gene, and even addition of whole extra chromosomes, can lead to serious clinical consequences such as Down's syndrome due to an extra copy of chromosome 21.

Avoid:

- Don't list all the mutations you can think of in no particular order
  - This question is looking for a structured response to show you understand the processes
- Don't expand too much on the consequences of RNA and DNA being longer or shorter; or how mutations arise, this is not relevant to the question
  - How RNA and DNA molecules code for proteins is not really relevant to this answer.

Q38: I can see from your personal statement that you do a lot of sports. What effects does lactic acid have on the body and brain?

What is this question exploring: This question is not only testing knowledge of physiology and the effects of lactic acid but an understanding of why these processes occur. It is not necessary to know all the detail or specific biochemistry of lactic acid's effects but pinpointing the main processes and speculating additional functions will demonstrate critical thinking and analysis.

Tips for a good answer:

- Explain why the processes you are describing occur in the body and brain
  - An awareness of physiological processes such as aerobic and anaerobic metabolism, and the way muscle cells function, will help to show a more integrative understanding of the effects of lactic acid
- Don't worry about not knowing specific biochemistry, especially neurophysiology
  - The specific chemistry of the effects of lactic acid in the brain is complicated and not necessary for this question. Use first principles of cells in an abnormal (acidic) environment, and how this may affect the processes occurring, to speculate.

- Despite the introductory statement, this question is not just asking about what happens during intense physical exercise and sport
  - Lactic acid can be implicated in other situations, often pathologically. Demonstrating this knowledge shows thinking outside of the box and not just following exactly what the interviewer has said.
- Link the answer to clinical situations
  - For example: lactic acidosis

Model answer: The demands of muscle tissue during strenuous exercise increase, meaning that aerobic demands exceed oxygen delivery to the tissues. Anaerobic metabolism must therefore aid the generation of energy through glycolysis where pyruvate is generated, and then converted to lactate, allowing energy production to continue. This can only continue for a short period of time but is necessary to allow energy production in high demand. The lactic acid produced by this process increases the acidity in muscle cells, which disrupts metabolism and other processes due to a suboptimal pH environment. Although this is in theory a negative effect, it prevents damage in high energy demand by slowing down muscle contractions. Lactate may travel in the systemic circulation to other tissues or be present in other tissues due to a decrease in the tissue's oxygen supply. The lactic acid generated from anaerobic metabolism in these cases can have a deleterious effect, including in the brain. Generally, the body's pH sits at a slightly alkaline level, optimum pH for the processes occurring in cells and enzymatic reactions. When this is disrupted, there can be severe effects including cell death, due to an imbalance of hydrogen ions in the environment disrupting ion gradients and cellular processes.

Avoid:

- Explaining physiology without explaining *why*
- Too much detail about why lactic acid forms while exercising
  - This is good extra knowledge but not what the question is asking

Q39: Why do bats and moles have different brain to body ratios?

What is this question exploring: This question is asking you to use critical thinking about a topic you may have little knowledge about. It is necessary to think about what the brain : body ratio may signify physiologically, and what this may have to do with specific species and their functions. Consider the different functions of a mole and bat, and what attributes they might need to fulfil these functions.

Tips for a good answer:

- Describe what the brain : body ratio may tell you about an animal
  - o Why might having a larger brain compared to body size, or vice versa, be beneficial evolutionarily?
  - o Specific knowledge of neuroanatomy is not necessary, however a demonstration of understanding about neurons and brain matter, and the main areas of the brain, may help here.
- Talk about evolution and natural selection
  - o Everything is specifically adapted for a particular function, and it is important to demonstrate this understanding when explaining why animals have certain anatomy or physiology
- It is not necessary to know (even vaguely!) the ratio for these two species, this is testing critical thinking and comparison

Model answer: Generally, brain size increases with body size, however, this is not a linear relationship. It may be thought that a higher brain : body ratio indicates a higher level of cognition, because the mass of neurons and brain matter may confer an ability to perform more diverse and complex tasks, however, this is not a direct correlation. It is very difficult to quantify 'intelligence', particularly between species; especially as certain layers or areas of the brain may be more important in quantifiable cognitive function than others (for example, the cerebral cortex). Both bats and moles are mammals, however, they serve very different functions in their environmental niche. Moles live a subterranean lifestyle, with little necessity for visual processing or other complex senses. Bats are nocturnal, meaning their vision is also poorly developed. On the other hand, they emit ultrasonic sounds for echolocation at different frequencies, which may require a different neural structure and potentially increased brain mass to process. Equally, bats are flying mammals, meaning that their body mass ratio may have evolved to be reduced (where brain mass may have remained to serve these specific functions) to make them lighter and more mobile in flight.

Avoid:

- Don't panic about not knowing anything about mole and bat brains
  - It is more impressive to an interviewer to work something out on first principles. Even if it is not necessarily exactly right, a point with a logical background will demonstrate thinking on the spot.
- Jumping into facts about the specific species without properly linking this to the question

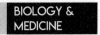

Q40: Please draw as many compounds as possible using C4H8O, placing emphasis on the different chemical groups involved.

What this question is exploring: This question is attempting to understand your knowledge of chemistry. It is relatively simple and draws upon knowledge of structural isomers and functional groups.

Tips for a good answer:

- Be methodical
  - o Instead of just writing as many as you can down split it up into categories e.g. functional group, structural isomer
- Start with easy first
  - o Don't overcomplicate things, start simple and then get more creative
- Keep going!
  - o You probably won't get every single one but keep going and think about the different shapes the carbon atoms can be rearranged into e.g. cyclical structures, double bonds
- Take this opportunity to show off! When talking about the different functional groups take the opportunity to talk about their different properties and reactions.

Model answer: First I'm going to look at all the different functional groups this structure could contain. I am going to make a table and sort the molecules by functional group. Then I will add molecules with different structures to the table.

(see table overleaf)

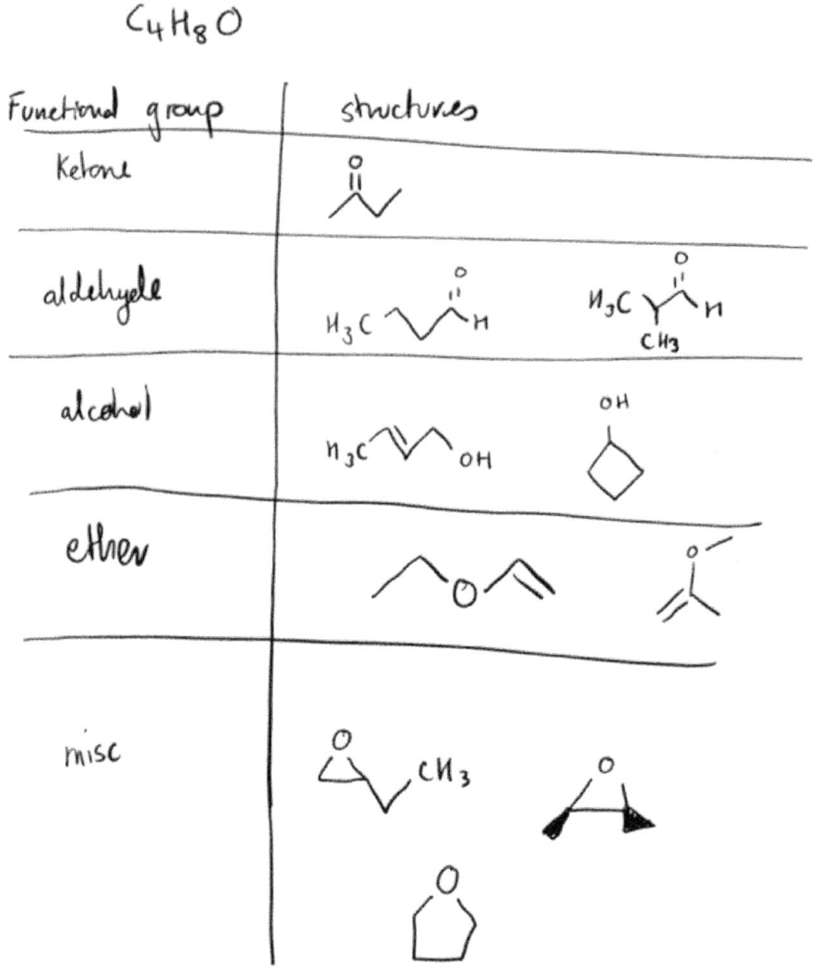

C_4H_8O

Functional group	structures
Ketone	
aldehyde	
alcohol	
ether	
misc	

Avoid:

- Drawing every molecule in a random order without explaining
- Not speaking to the interviewer about your thought process - it is important they can understand what you are thinking

Q41: What do you know about the bonding in a benzene ring?

You are expected to know about the structure and bonding of benzene from your A-levels. A question which simply asks 'what do you know' may seem so open ended that you're unsure where to begin. However, it is worth bearing in mind that your interviewers will prompt you with extra information or questions if you say something which they'd like you to explore further, and so if you simply start by summarising facts you may soon find that you have a lot more to say than you initially realised.

Although you should avoid spending too much time in your interview worrying about why they're asking you a question, it can be useful to consider the context at least a little in order to prioritise the information in your answer. Your knowledge that benzene rings are active in a number of pharmaceutical compounds may help in the later stages of this question.

A **poor applicant** may be unfamiliar with benzene due to poor preparation for their interview. Alternatively, they may give a particularly short or closed answer such as "benzene is a hexagon of 6 carbons and the hydrogens attached", and then fail to elaborate further even under further prompting.

An **average applicant** would state facts from memory based on their studies at school. For example, "Benzene is C_6H_6. It involves a delocalised cloud of electrons, which is why there are only 6 bonded hydrogens, rather than the 12 you'd find in a molecule such as cyclohexane". They may also comment on the molecular shape or bonding angles.

A **good applicant** would build on their explanation of the structure to begin to link structure to chemical properties, or perhaps even uses. They may also discuss ways in which molecules containing benzene are categorised as aromatic rather than aliphatic compounds, and why this distinction arose. This is where you can really distinguish your understanding and set yourself apart from those candidates who only know 'the basics'. For example, where are the delocalised electrons found in the structure (in terms of s or p orbitals)? How do the delocalised electrons contribute to the stability of the molecule?

Excellent applicants would be able to link this increased energetic stability as well as the solubility and volatility of benzene and many of its derivatives to their pharmaceutical applications. Importantly, the candidate may not *know* what the links are, but would be able to make intelligent suggestions. For example, 'as benzene is a relatively small molecule, it may be more easily absorbed in the lungs or small intestine'.

Q42: An ice cube is floating in a glass of water. What happens to the water level when it melts?

This question is a relatively common scientific brain teaser, and as such, is unlikely to arise in an actual interview due to the risk that too many applicants are unfairly advantaged by having seen it before. That being said, it demonstrates a number of key skills which you will need to develop in your interview preparation, and aims to test your ability to logically reason your way through a somewhat confusing situation based on relatively basic scientific knowledge.

A **poor applicant** may simply state an answer – "the water level will rise/fall/stay the same". They have in this case a one in three chance of having guessed the correct answer. If they haven't explained a thought process that they used to work out the answer, even if that thought process was there internally, the interviewer has no way of knowing whether they actually worked this out at all or simply guessed, and as a result they would gain no credit.

A **good applicant** may begin their answer with their gut instinct 'I think the water level would rise', for example, and although this isn't necessary, it isn't inherently harmful either. The *must* then go on to logically reason their way through to a justification for their answer, and shouldn't be afraid of changing their mind in the face of evidence which contradicts their initial statement.

In this case, it is important to first highlight Archimedes' principle, and the idea of buoyancy based on the displacement of water. In short, when the ice is floating in the glass, there will be enough ice below the surface of the water to displace a mass of water equal to the mass of the ice cube. Although it is fairly intuitive to state that ice would float with some of it's volume above and some below the water's surface, the candidate should justify this by explaining whether ice or water are more dense.

Following this, it is important to consider whether the melted ice cube would take up a smaller, larger, or the same volume as the mass of water which was displaced when it was ice. Given that the displaced volume was such that the mass of water displaced equalled the mass of the ice, the ice will, when melted, take up the exact same volume. As a result, the water level would remain the same following the melting of the ice.

Some students find this easier to visualise in reverse, instead considering what would happen if water was removed from a glass, frozen, and added back in.

Although you may not get all the way through to a final answer without prompting, as long as you have shown a logical synthesis of your pre-existing knowledge with the context of the question you've been asked you will have given a successful answer.

Q43: How is aspirin synthesised?

Although it is relatively unusual for questions to simply ask you to recap your knowledge from your A-level (or equivalent) studies, your scientific knowledge, preparation, and general competence is important. When targeting your preparation for the interview it is therefore important to revise (or even read ahead) on your chemistry studies, and take a particular focus on anything which has a clear medical relevance, such as the synthesis of pharmaceutical compounds like aspirin.

It's important to remember that this shouldn't be a 'chore'. As an aspiring medic, you should, hopefully, be interested in learning more about *why* medicines work the way they do, and *how* they interact with the systems in the human body. So asking these questions as you work through your chemistry (and biology) studies is hopefully something that you will be doing for your own interest, rather than simply to 'tick a box' for your application.

If you haven't encountered aspirin before, or have forgotten, it is likely that the interviewers would provide a chemical structure of aspirin, such as the one below, in order to help start your thinking:

A **poor applicant** may struggle to identify any ways in which aspirin may be synthesised, even with the help of the chemical structure.

An **average applicant** may be able to break down the structure of the molecule (for example identifying that the ester link means that there is likely an esterification step) into some steps, either from memory or logical deduction. They may struggle to answer follow up questions from the interviewers such as 'why would we need these conditions in this step?' or 'what does this step achieve?' – particularly if their summary is based on memorisation of their school work rather than the deeper level of understanding.

Good applicants would be able to summarise the steps in the synthesis of aspirin, including:

- The reaction of ethanoic anhydride with salicylic acid
- The use of a sulfuric acid catalyst
- The reaction taking place under reflux, with the aspirin then condensed out

They would also offer reasonable explanations or suggestions for the further questions the interviewer may ask – for example why is an anhydride used rather than an alcohol? Importantly, they needn't know the answer to these before the interview, but should be able to make suggestions, for example is the anhydride likely to be more or less reactive than an alcohol would be?

Q44: Draw the full chemical structure of DNA.

This question would most likely form the beginning of a longer discussion about any of a number of topics related to the structure of DNA and its function. However, even as a standalone question, there is a lot of opportunity for the interviewer to ask questions throughout the process relating to a wide range of medically relevant topical research issues, for example cancer development, CRISPR, and other genetic engineering.

A **poor applicant** may be able to recall some of the basics of DNA structure, for example the double helix formed by the strands, with A, T, C and G base pairs throughout. However, they may be unsure of any more detail than this, or may have forgotten key definitions (for example, what are A, T, C, and G?). As a result, they will be unable to use their structure as the basis for any of the more advanced questions they may be asked.

An **average applicant** will be able to name the four bases, as well as drawing the detail of each of the sugar-phosphate 'backbone' of each of the strands of DNA. They may not be able to link the structure they have drawn to the full name of DNA, or be able to answer questions on how the bonding between each of the molecules would introduce areas of weakness, or allow for processes such as translation or transcription.

A **good applicant** will not only be aware of what each component of the molecule is, but will also be able to discuss the bonding within the molecule. As an example, the differences in bonding between base pairs, as a result of the structure of each of the bases, should be incorporated or discussed as part of their diagram.

You should expect this to be the minimum acceptable level of knowledge upon which the interviewers would base further questioning. As a result, it's not only important to be able to recall the structure of DNA but also identify the importance of each of the different parts of the structure to the molecules characteristic behaviour. As you're working through your biology and chemistry preparation, make sure to ask *why* things work, rather than just accepting they do.

Q45: Why are diamonds so valuable?

This question might seem as though it would be a discussion more suited to an economics interview than a medical one. However it asks candidates to link their academic knowledge in chemistry to real-world situations. And given cost considerations are common constraints, particularly in questions more focussed on medical ethics, having an understanding of basic economics is no bad thing regardless!

A **poor candidate** may consider supply and demand but give a relatively superficial answer such as: "there isn't very much of it, so it costs more" or "people like the way it looks so they're happy to pay more for it". This, however, fails to address the two key points of the question – firstly, why is this true of *diamond* and not other (similarly scarce or in demand) materials, and secondly, what do we even mean by *valuable* at all?

Although the question doesn't ask anything about structure or bonding, it is important for all candidates to understand that as the properties, and therefore uses and value of materials, are determined by their structure and bonding, this is an important starting point.

A **good candidate** may answer one, but not both of these questions. For example, they may talk about properties of diamond which make it useful for a range of applications, such as its strength, lack of reactivity, or ease of extraction. They may then link these properties to the wide range of uses which diamonds have as a result, such as in high precision cutting tools.

Alternatively, they may give an answer which asks more questions than it answers, contains minor areas in which it is factually incorrect, or argues which gold shouldn't be that valuable after all: "diamonds are relatively easy to extract because they aren't reactive, and they're generally used for non-essential purposes such as jewellery". While many of the points being made here are interesting, unless they are explored further this answer would be incomplete.

The **best candidates** would give an answer which demonstrates their clear knowledge of the material properties which makes diamonds useful and in-demand. They would then go on to attempt to answer the seemingly contradictory questions about economic value, for example, if it is easier to extract than other materials why isn't it cheaper? The important thing is that the interviewer isn't looking for anything complex in terms of economic theory, but they're also not looking for an unjustified dismissive comment such as "people are conned into thinking it's worth something" either.

Q46: What is entropy?

This is another question which is testing your interview preparation, and would likely form an introduction to a more advanced discussion of your thought process surrounding the meaning of or consequences of entropy. Nonetheless, it is important to be able to give a good answer which shows that you understand the meaning of what you've been taught, and haven't just remembered key facts or statements to say. Similarly, you need to be able to give an answer which is concise and succinct, without being so short that the interviewers have nothing to comment on or ask you questions about (or so short it seems like you've not understood the topic fully).

Poor answers may indicate that the candidate hasn't really understood what entropy is, or is describing a related (but different) concept such as enthalpy. Alternatively, the candidate may simply state they're unsure of how to explain their answer, and give a very limited answer as a result.

Perhaps surprisingly, a common mistake in **average answers** comes from students attempting to show they understand entropy completely. It's important to bear in mind that there are some concepts (such as entropy) which are just *difficult* to conceptualise. As a result, appearing overconfident, or even arrogant, about how simple the concept is, is unlikely to convey what the applicant is intending. It will instead, generally, communicate that they don't have a full grasp of just how nuanced or complex the topic actually is – the exact opposite of their intention. There is, therefore, a difficult balance to strike here.

Good answers will include any, or all of the following entropy ideas:

- Entropy is, in summary, a measure of the tendency of a system to become more disordered or random.
- There is a link, demonstrated by the equation $\Delta G = \Delta H - T\Delta S$, between entropy, enthalpy, and the likelihood of spontaneous reaction. Candidates should be able to define all the terms in their reactions.

It is likely that this would lead to further exploration of the meaning of 'spontaneous' reaction, or calculations of the temperatures at which certain reactions would take place. The candidate may then be asked to draw conclusions about why certain biological processes occur at certain temperatures, or why certain chemicals are safe in humans despite high levels of reactivity in other scenarios. The key to success here is, as noted in previous questions, in ensuring you examine *why* things work the way they do when you're learning them, rather than considering the question of 'why' for the first time when your Oxbridge interviewer asks you!

Q47: Why are bacterial infections easier to treat than viral infections?

Given the relatively recent events surrounding the covid-19 pandemic applicants will be expected to not only understand the basic biological concepts, but also be able to apply them to real-world scenarios or challenges.

Though it may sound obvious, it is important prior to answering any interview question to ensure you're fully clear on the exact question you're answering. Many **poor answers** to this question revolve around a summary of the differences between bacteria and viruses. Although this is a useful starting point, if a candidate doesn't use this to answer the question about ease of treatment, they will be given little credit. Questions about the differences in structure, prevention, and treatment, could all arise – so make sure you're clear on exactly which aspect you need to be focussing on before you start your answer.

A **good answer** would begin by summarising the infection mechanisms which viruses and bacteria employ, as well as the key differences between them. Although this, again may seem only tangentially related to the question, it is an important starting point from which the treatment options can be explored. The answer would then move on to link the different infection mechanisms to the difficulties in treating virus-borne illnesses rather than bacterial illnesses, as a result of the potential damage to the host cells.

An **excellent answer** may also include a description of the exact mechanisms by which antibacterial drugs work, for example in targeting areas of the cell which are common across a range of bacteria, rather than areas specific to individual strains of viruses.

Importantly, though it may be tempting to bring in knowledge of preventative measures which can be taken to target infections, the focus on treatment means this should be your primary concern. You're not expected to be experts in virology, but you would hopefully have given some consideration to the question 'how does the treatment for covid work?' or 'why are scientists unable to create a cure for covid?', which you can then extrapolate from for viral infections in general.

Q48: Does the molecular structure of glycine change with pH?

Although your preparation for the interview (and your A-levels) would hopefully mean you understood at least the basics of amino acids, your interviewers would be likely to provide you with a diagram of glycine to ensure that you had the information you needed to be able to make reasonable deductions:

A **poor answer** may struggle to identify any areas of the molecule which would be affected by pH changes or give a vague or noncommittal answer such as "the structure would change because the hydrogens would increase or decrease". Although this is not strictly incorrect, it doesn't show a precise understanding of where on the molecule would be influenced and may seem to an interviewer like the candidate is trying to 'hedge their bets' without a full understanding.

An **average answer** may explain how the structure would change with a change of pH in one direction (for example, with a low pH), but then fail to consider the effect of the opposite change. They would therefore have displayed their understanding of some of the key concepts being tested but would have given an incomplete answer. It's therefore important that you always try to end your answer by returning to the original question to check you've answered fully.

A **good answer** would be able to identify the different regions of the molecule which would be affected and summarise what the molecule would look like in high and low pH. It may also propose how those changes in pH would be achieved or summarise which reactions might take place as a result.

The **strongest answers** would show an understanding of the concept of zwitterions and be able to explain the way in which amino acids can function as both proton donors and proton acceptors simultaneously. They would also (perhaps as a result of prompting by the interviewer) begin to link this to some of the behaviours in biological systems.

Q49: How long is a gene? Why are genes the length they are?

It is relatively uncommon, though not impossible, for the question you're asked at interview to be relatively closed-ended, such as this question. At first glance, this can seem incredibly challenging, because surely you either *know* or you can't answer. It's important to remember that even in questions like this one they're not expecting you to simply recall the average length of a gene. Instead, you can use your knowledge of how genes are composed to gradually work towards an estimated answer. Importantly, your final estimate might be completely incorrect, but as long as you've stated your assumptions, and used reasonable and justified values, that will not affect the strength of your answer at all.

A **poor applicant** might struggle, even if supported by the interviewer, to know where to start with this question. This is often due to a fear of beginning an answer without a plan for how your method will develop to give you the answer you need. However, it's important to remember that this is not what the interviewers are looking for, and so even explaining areas of uncertainty would be a starting point.

A **good applicant** would perhaps begin by summarising what genes do, and how their structure can be broken down into codons and bases. The very shortest genes can be only a few hundred bases long.

At this point, the interviewer may prompt the candidate to move onto the secondary question, or why genes have the length they do.

At this point, the **best applicants** may be able to bring in their advanced knowledge of the functions of genes (including non-coding genes) in order to propose an explanation. While knowledge of areas of genetic code such as introns isn't assumed knowledge, it is a good idea to ensure you have a passing understanding of what they are and why they haven't been removed by natural selection given their lack of direct benefit.

Q50: How many genes are in a cell?

As with the previous question, this question could in theory be answered with a single quoted value if it is a piece of information you happen to know. However, as mentioned previously it is perfectly possible to give an excellent answer without ever giving a numerical answer, and similarly possible to give a particularly poor answer which does include a lucky guess of the correct answer.

A **poor candidate** would, again, struggle to give an answer, or even form an idea of where to start based on their attempts to give a single numerical answer. Alternatively they may state basic genetic information, for example 'there are 23 chromosome pairs per cell' but fail to link this to anything which works towards an answer to the question.

A **good candidate** may recognise that the interviewer is unlikely to be looking for an exact answer (e.g. '20', '20,000' or '20,000,000') and instead will be hoping for a discussion around the magnitude of the solution instead.

The correct answer Is 25-35 thousand genes in the average human cell, however, even if the applicant were to guess a much higher number (or give no number at all), there are a few key points they could make to prompt further discussion. For example:

- What do genes do?
- Are there the same number of genes in all cells?
- Does the number of genes in a cell vary with time?
- If genes code for proteins, would knowledge of the number of proteins used in the human body help deduce an answer?

This final point is one of the most important to a successful Oxbridge interview. **Excellent candidates** will often fail to reach an answer, but instead give a solution which states, 'if I had this information and this information, then I would be able to deduce the answer by doing…'. Being able to identify which information would help you derive the answer, and demonstrate your ability to approach unfamiliar situations by asking intelligent questions is a valuable skill.

Q51: Give an example of when specialist biological knowledge has helped a global issue.

This question is reflective of many of the 'ice-breaker' or introductory questions which you may be faced with earlier in the interview. It's important to note that there is no right answer, and that many Oxbridge interviews won't have these types of questions (or questions about your personal statement, interests, or motivations) because many of the tutors like to focus on more technical scientifical or mathematical questions.

In preparing for these types of questions it is therefore important to understand *why* they are asked at all, and there are two main reasons to consider here. Firstly, and perhaps most obviously, they allow you to show your interest in and motivation for the subject, as well as any evidence of your wider reading. However, if you're applying to study your subject at Oxbridge, the interviewers can probably operate on the assumption that the vast majority of candidates will have this motivation, and so this is not a distinguishing factor. The primary reason for asking questions such as these at the start of an interview must, then, be something different. Their main purpose is simply to get you talking. You will likely be nervous in your interview, no matter how well you've prepared, and therefore asking you to talk about yourself or your interests is one of the best ways to get you talking about something 'easy', before they lead into the technical questions. You should use them as an opportunity to get the conversation with the interviewers off to a start, and ease yourself into the interview as much as possible, which will make it easier for you to clearly explain your answers when you're doing the later, and likely more important, questions because you'll already have broken the silence.

There are still *wrong* ways to answer this question. A **poor answer** would show little knowledge of even a single development in the field; or perhaps little understanding of where specialist knowledge was applied within a given advance. It's also important not to try and be too unique here – some students every year insist on trying to find a topic to talk about which their interviewers won't have heard of, in the hopes of seeming well read. However, it's much more important to give a sensible (if common) answer, than one which no one else has given because it's demonstrably less important than others which you appear to have overlooked.

A **good answer** would summarise both the example you're including, as well as how it helped a global issue.

There are a wide range of examples and justifications which could be used, you may wish to consider an example which overcame a particularly tricky biological challenge (for example the development of a cure for HIV), or an example which overcame a particularly difficult social challenge (for example the speed required for the development of the covid vaccine).

Importantly, there are a range of related questions (e.g. 'what do you think is the most important recent advancement in medicine?' or 'can you give an example of some research you've read which you found particularly interesting?') which could be asked. It is good practice to have a well-rehearsed example which you can adapt for any of these questions. This will also be helpful at any other medical schools you're applying for, particularly those in which you'll be doing MMIs.

Q52: Was Lamarck right?

This question aims to test your understanding of the theory of Lamarckian evolution, as well as your wider reading and knowledge of currently topical recent areas such as epigenetics. Importantly, you should demonstrate a comprehensive method of the scientific method: hypothesis, evidence, and theory. You should also ensure that you show an understanding of the strengths and weaknesses of the iterative nature of the scientific method.

If an applicant didn't understand or remember the concepts of Lamarckian evolution, the interviewer may begin by giving a brief summary such as: "The theory proposed by Lamarck, prior to Darwin's theory of evolution by natural selection, suggested that organisms would pass on adaptations they'd individually acquired throughout their lifetime to their offspring. For example, if a giraffe stretched its neck throughout its lifetime in order to reach higher branches, it would then pass this onto its offspring."

A **poor applicant** may struggle to give an answer, even with the prompting and explanation above, or fail link any evidence to the arguments for or against the theory. They may also fail to give a balanced explanation. Given that the question is about whether Lamarck was right, it should be assumed that an answer as simple as 'no' is somewhat missing the point, and care should be taken to justify arguments made.

A **good applicant** would be able to give an answer which shows an understanding of the way in which science develops, and an awareness that it would be pointless to judge the ability of scientists over 200 years ago, who were working with considerably different equipment, by todays knowledge.

The **best applicants** will be able to link the theory of Lamarckian evolution to current advances in the field such as epigenetic mutation. This is the idea that environmentally influenced mutations can be acquired and cause genetic changes which are then inherited by offspring. (A widely researched example of this is in the predisposition to mental health conditions such as anxiety in the descendants of Holocaust survivors). However, they will also temper this with a clear understanding of the fact that research into epigenetic mutation is still largely in its infancy, and as a result any conclusions drawn are likely to complement Darwinian evolution rather than 'rewriting the text books'.

Q53: How would you mass produce insulin?

This question highlights a key concept in the area of medical research – the synthetic replication of biological processes. In short, applicants should have an awareness that the most effective ways to replicate biological processes is often to recreate the process using biological materials, rather than attempting to artificially synthesise compounds from scratch. Whether or not this is a topic which you have previously encountered or discussed, applicants should be able to propose sensible ways in which mass production could be achieved.

A **poor candidate** may give a vague or noncommittal answer such as "you'd need to analyse the structure of insulin, and then figure out how to recreate the reactions that happen in the pancreas outside the body". Although this is, in some ways, correct – the question is looking for suggestions as to how those reactions could be recreated rather than a simple statement that they would need to be. As a result, the interviewers would likely prompt for further development, and give little credit to an answer which stopped here.

A **good candidate** may focus more on ways in which the biological processes could be directly copied, rather than artificially synthesised, given this is a common method. For example, could insulin producing cells be cultured in a growth medium and used to produce insulin. What would the limitations of this approach be? Alternatively, candidates may suggest examples of research in related fields which they may be familiar with from their wider reading. For example, the development of genetically engineered goats which produce milk with a high insulin content which can then be extracted and purified for use in drugs.

The **best candidates** will firstly be able to suggest ways in which mass production could be achieved. For example, instead of using human cells, the insulin producing genes could be inserted into cells with a much higher replication rate such as bacteria in order to grow more insulin producing cells in a shorter time, and therefore increase yield. They may also attempt to explain why using a method such as the one above is simpler, easier, or more successful than artificial synthesis, perhaps with reference to the chirality of a number of common biological molecules, and the issues this poses for purification.

Q54: How would you tell if a mouse could differentiate between the smell of an apple and the smell of chocolate?

Questions in which applicants are asked to develop their own experimental methods are not uncommon in Oxbridge interviews. This is because they require you to apply your existing knowledge to an unfamiliar or hypothetical scenario, as well as demonstrating your understanding of key principles of medical research and the fundamentals of the scientific method. It is important to logically approach the question, perhaps beginning by defining basic experimental concepts such as the independent, dependent, and control variables, particularly if you were struggling to know where to begin.

Poor applicants will often operate on the assumption that there is a single right answer, or that they are being asked to quote from an experiment they should remember from school. As a result they can be easily thrown off course, and can find it challenging in questions such as this one in which there are many solutions which could be correct provided they were well justified and explored.

Good applicants will be able to propose a hypothesis, and then develop a method by which mice would be tested for their response to the smells of chocolate and apple. Importantly, they would identify the way in which they would be able to tell if the mice were capable of differentiating, as well as identifying potential flaws. For example, "we would be able to tell that they could differentiate if they exposed a preference for one of the smells over the other based on whether they appeared to prefer chocolate or apples". However, there are issues in this, such as "one problem is that this depends on the mice preferring one of the rewards, and so if the mice liked both rewards equally then even if they were differentiating we might not be able to tell if they selected each smell equally". The candidate could then propose a solution (e.g. associating one of the smells with a reward and one with a 'punishment') which could be employed to overcome this issue.

The **best applicants** would build on this and incorporate methods for ensuring the significance of the results, such as repeated testing, the use of control groups, or links with other research into similar smells. They may then engage in a discussion with the interviewer on follow up questions such as 'how can the mouse differentiate between the smells?' which are testing an entirely different skill set.

Q55: Should all stem cell therapy be legalised?

This question is one of a number of different 'ethically challenging' questions which could be asked in a medical interview (other examples could include provision of abortion, euthanasia, life-support, or certain mental health treatments). It is therefore in your interest when preparing to develop an outline of a method which you can apply to all questions of this type in order to reliably and logically structure your answer, incorporating your own knowledge, opposing viewpoints, and pillars of medical ethics into a rigorous conclusion. An example of such an outline may be something like:

- Begin with a summary of the context (e.g. what is stem cell therapy?)
- Consider arguments in favour (medical, social, economic)
- Consider arguments against (using the same broad categories as above)
- Link to the pillars of medical ethics using at least one example
- Draw a conclusion

A **poor answer** to this question would therefore fail to show a consideration of opposing viewpoints, or understanding of both sides. In many cases it is natural that as a scientifically-focussed aspiring medic you will favour empirical research, however statements such as "there's no good reason to oppose stem cell research" show an inability to understand or empathise with different people's belief systems, which will not be well received. Empathy and non-judgemental communication are both essential skills of good doctors (just consider how many doctors must be able to successfully engage with and allay the fears of members of the public who are against vaccination).

A **good answer** would be balanced, with at least one argument for and against. Importantly, you should try to begin with an indication of how you are going to conclude your argument, for example "Yes, I believe all stem cell therapies could be legalised. The main reasoning for this is…. However, there are arguments made against legalisation and these are…". Many students interpret 'balanced response' as description of arguments for followed by description of arguments against. However, you should be analysing the arguments at each step, and it shouldn't be a surprise to the interviewer which conclusion you come to at the end! Being able to balance this ability to put together a coherent and easily understandable answer, while still making sure it's balanced and as unbiased as possible is a difficult skill to master, and so practice is essential.

The **best answers** would pick out key areas of nuance within the question, as well as incorporating specific named medical ethics frameworks, rather than more vague statements about 'ensuring doctors act ethically'. For example, the question refers to multiple types of stem cell therapy, and so some answers may consider whether some are more or less justifiable then others.

Q56: If senses work only because our brain interprets electrical signals, what is reality?

Although rare, this somewhat stereotypical Oxbridge interview question, being philosophical and hypothetical in nature could still arise. Most applicants struggle with questions like this based on how different they are from questions styles which they've practiced answering. A good technique for approaching questions which you're unsure of is to buy yourself a little bit of time by summarising or defining key terms. For example, if you're struggling to identify ways to give a logical response to this question, instead begin by attempting to summarise how senses work, and then move on to attempt to define 'reality' and before you know it you'll be working through the difficult areas of the question!

A **poor answer** to this question would show a lack of awareness of the uncertainty of the issue at hand. Some applicants, in an attempt to demonstrate their grasp of scientific concepts, can inadvertently give the impression that they believe all questions have a single correct answer. For example, they may say "reality is the external stimuli which we all interact with and which is the same for all of us – how our brain works is completely irrelevant to this, because it's just a question of what is in the universe". While this may seem reassuringly certain, humility and an awareness that there are some things which are either unknown or unknowable are essential skills for good doctors.

Good answers will therefore primarily highlight areas for discussion within the question – either giving several competing areas, or one example explored in detail. There is no right answer to this question! For example, could "I think, therefore I am" be extended to "I think it is, therefore it is"? Alternatively, applicants may avoid a philosophical approach in favour of a more direct biological or medical approach – can we learn about the meaning of reality by exploring the similarities and differences in experiences between people with differently functioning senses? What data could we gain from this 'experiment'?

The **best answers** might consider whether the underlying assumption of the question – that the electrical signals themselves aren't reality – is justified. Clearly our brain is capable of influencing our reality, as shown by the placebo and nocebo affect, as well as in optical illusions and other examples. If this is the case, is there a single unified reality? Or is reality individual to each person?

Q57: How many guinea pigs would you use in an experiment?

The use of animal testing in the development of medical treatments is a commonly arising medical ethics question. As with previous medical ethics questions, it is important to consider arguments for and against the practice within the context of the pillars of medical ethics which doctors (and researchers in the field) will aim to uphold. Importantly, this question isn't asking whether animal testing is justifiable, it's asking how many animals you would test on in an experiment, and therefore you should ensure that you don't use a 'one-size-fits-all' approach and answer a different question than the one asked.

A **poor answer** may simply identify pros and cons of the use of guinea pigs, or spend too much time trying to create a specific answer, e.g. "I'd use 50", without exploring their assumptions or logically working their way through the question.

A **good answer** would begin with a brief summary of the issue at hand, and very quickly turn to answering this specific question. A primary consideration which the applicant should discuss is 'what is the experiment?'. It is impossible to determine how many test subjects, and what type of test subject, would be valuable without knowing more about the experiment being carried out. For example, in phase III trials, the aim is to compare a newly developed drug with the existing treatment and compare efficacy and side effects in human test subjects. In this case, the correct answer would be 0, so further detail is clearly needed.

The **best answers** would therefore begin to develop a framework for the types of questions which would need to be asked to determine the number for a wide range of experiments. For example, the following would all be good questions to propose: What is the statistical significance required? Is the experiment aiming to determine lethal dosage or simply compare side effects? How many previous trials have taken place, and how similar is the new therapy to the existing options?

The inherent uncertainty in scientific experimentation, and the requirement for multiple tests to ensure reliability and replicability would be another excellent point to include in a top-level answer.

Q58: Is euthanasia too broad a term to use? What are the different types of euthanasia?

As one of the key medical discussions of the last few years, you should, as an aspiring medic, be incredibly familiar with arguments for and against expanding access to or legalising euthanasia. You should also, ideally, be aware of related medical issues, such as the issues with the Liverpool Care Pathway for palliative care in the early 2010s.

A **poor answer** may show a limited or non-existent understanding of the meaning of euthanasia. Alternatively it may answer a different question such as 'what is euthanasia?' or 'what are the ethical arguments for and against euthanasia?'. While it can be easy to fall into the trap of giving an answer you've practiced previously, it is important that you ensure you answer the question you are asked, and not the one you prepared to be asked.

A **good answer** would give a definition of euthanasia, and be able to pull out some of the key differences between types of euthanasia. Even if you were unaware of types of euthanasia before the interview, you should be able to categorise different situations based on your understanding of times in which euthanasia may be appropriate. For example, assisted suicide general occurs when a person who typically is not about to die imminently is helped to die by medical professionals before a chronic or life-limiting illness progresses beyond a point they are comfortable with. This is clearly quite different to a situation in which a person who will die without significant medical intervention is allowed to die due to the medical intervention being withheld. This is different again to situations which are already more widely socially accepted for example the withdrawal of life support from individuals who will die without it.

An **excellent answer** may build on some of the examples given above in an attempt to categorise (e.g. into 'passive' v 'active' forms of euthanasia). They would then link this back to the first question asked – is euthanasia too broad a term? In order to answer this they would need to explore the value of having a term for any medical procedure, and then the issues which can arise if different people consider the term to mean different things due to a lack of specificity. Finally, they may, in discussion with their interviewers, begin to propose different ways in which social or medical acceptance of the different forms may be achieved, or explore whether certain types are more justifiable than others.

Q59: Should patients always have complete autonomy?

Before your interview you should have prepared for a question along the lines of 'why is [pillar of medical ethics] so important?'. As one of the four, it is likely that you will have a practiced answer relating to the importance and value of autonomy within healthcare provision. The challenge in this question is to apply your knowledge, and adapt the answer you have prepared in order to demonstrate your understanding of the grey areas surrounding patient autonomy.

A **poor answer** may be unfamiliar with, or unable to give an accurate definition of autonomy. Alternatively, it may be unbalanced, answering a simple 'yes' or 'no' without considering why this is a challenging question to answer, and the ways in which the ambiguity could be addressed.

A **good answer** would begin by defining autonomy and outlining its importance and the reason for its inclusion at the core of medical practice. It may then go on to use examples to demonstrate times in which it would be difficult to justify complete autonomy for patients. Recent examples from the Court of Protection are always worth being aware of (for example, there was a case in March 2020 in which the Court ordered that a man with learning difficulties, who was unable to make decisions for himself, was given the covid vaccination against the wishes of his family). A

The **best answers** would build on the case-by-case nature of the examples explored above in order to attempt to explain or justify generalised guidelines for situations in which autonomy must be limited. Importantly, they should show an understanding of situations in which autonomy may need to be limited, as well as situations in which a medical professional may restrict the autonomy of a patient incorrectly. Incorporating knowledge about good communication, informed consent, and the ways in which doctors can ensure that patient autonomy is respected in general would be valuable here too.

Q60: How much money should the NHS spend on palliative care?

Questions about the allocation of limited resources and budgets with public healthcare are also common at interview. It is important to strike a balance between avoiding giving a specific answer (it is unlikely you'll be able to justify the fact it should be exactly £3.752 billion, no matter how hard you try), while not being too vague. Many applicants fall into the trap of giving an answer which boils down to a statement that 'this is a very difficult question to try and answer'. While this is correct (and that's why they're asking you), simply acknowledging the difficulties is not enough, you should try to give specific and measurable ways in which those challenges could be quantified and overcome.

Additionally, in this question, you must be able to rely on your knowledge of what palliative care is, and the pros and cons of funding to public health.

Poor applicants may focus too heavily on trying to develop a specific value, and as a result lose sight of the bigger themes which need to be drawn out in the question. They may, alternatively, focus too heavily on one side of the debate (e.g. the pros or cons) in order to justify their answer, while failing to proactively acknowledge and incorporate challenges.

Good applicants will give a balanced account of the benefits and controversies surrounding the provision of palliative care. They will then move on to explore justifications for the NHS allocating a higher or lower proportion of its budget to such care, which should consider subtly different arguments to those mentioned previously.

The **best applicants** will use the range of discussion points mentioned above in order to draw a clear conclusion about the stance which they believe doctors and the NHS should take to palliative care. They may incorporate ideal traits into their answer. For example, while some doctors may argue against palliative care based on the idea that it simply prolongs the inevitable (see the development of the Liverpool Care Pathway as an example of this viewpoint) does that really embody a patient-centric approach? Can doctors be beneficent while discussing whether spending money on some end of life care is a waste? If not, how should this be addressed differently?

Q61: Why do some people describe the NHS as the 'crown jewel of the welfare state'?

Here the interviewers are looking to see if you have a basic understanding of the NHS, what its purpose is and how it functions. The question is clearly phrased to get you to discuss the positive aspects of the NHS: whilst it has a lot of flaws which you might want to mention, remember that this is also the institution that will fund half your studies, train you, and provide you with a job for your whole career (for the majority of you). Now is the time to show that you are not only passionate about medicine, but specifically your excitement of working in the UK and therefore for the NHS.

Good candidate: The NHS is undoubtedly one of the greatest achievements of the government in the realm of social care. The NHS is a source of immense pride for Briton's and for myself and I am very excited and indeed proud to (hopefully) eventually work for it. It provides some of the world's highest quality of care whilst providing it for free and more importantly, for all. It was set up in 1946 and is funded by general taxation hence it being free at the point of use. As per the founding principles of the White Paper, NHS services are available to all. The NHS has 7 key principles, which place the patient at the heart of its service, and bases access on clinical need and not on ability to pay. I think the non-discriminatory nature of access to the NHS is what makes it such a pride of the welfare state: other countries such as the US have incredibly high standards of care too, but its inaccessibility to the socio-economically deprived taints it. Although the NHS has undergone reforms since its foundation and is still far from perfect now, it continues to successfully provide high-quality and free services for everyone who needs it, which is not something that can be said for all other parts of the welfare state (such as education or certain social services) – this is why it may be considered the crown jewel.

This answer demonstrates knowledge on the founding principles of the NHS and shows enthusiasm for your future employer. Acknowledging faults in the system shows you are not naïve either, but it is important to recognise the enormity of the NHS and its successes in continuing to provide services despite being overstretched and underfunded etc.

A poor candidate may just address the fact that its free to everyone but without really qualifying this statement and explaining why that makes it such a success. They might not use this opportunity to flash any extra knowledge from reading or to demonstrate any enthusiasm.

Q62: How well can we compare public and private healthcare?

This question is tricky because it requires you to really think about what is being asked of you. It would be really easy to fall into a trap of arguing for or against private healthcare and giving your opinion on the morality of it, however this isn't what the question is asking. What is actually being alluded to is whether or not there is any point in comparing these two forms of healthcare – do they serve such different purposes that you would be comparing apples and oranges? One strategy to approach this might be to begin comparing them, and then seeing how relevant it is to weigh up one against the other, or whether actually it is possible to have both because they fill different gaps in society.

Good applicant: Public and private healthcare could be directly compared to each other in terms of cost, access to services, waiting times, patient autonomy and arguably to quality of care. However, it is not necessarily useful nor appropriate to do so. Comparing them implies there is a choice to be made between the two; that the two could fill the same niche. In the UK, private healthcare serves a very different purpose to the NHS. Public healthcare in the UK is based on the fundamental principle that access to services is based on clinical need and not on financial status. Private healthcare works on the principle that money opens up faster access to more services and (to an extent) a greater degree of comfort. But to compare them by judging them against the same standards is unfair given that they run off different principles and it is unrealistic to expect a publicly, tax funded system that serves (more than) an entire population to have the same priorities as one aimed at a smaller population of the wealthy. There are also some services only offered by one or the other – for example emergency services are only really provided by the NHS, whereas cosmetic work is largely private healthcare.

In conclusion, many of the outcomes of both healthcare systems could be compared, but given the different priorities of the two systems, I would argue any comparison drawn would not be valid. As they don't play the same role in UK society and they are not two ways of doing the same thing, it doesn't make much sense to compare them.

Whatever your opinion on the matter is, a good candidate will answer the question carefully and by considering actually what both public and private healthcare aim to do for society and therefore what outcomes you could measure in both.

A bad applicant would not engage with the question and misinterpret the question by answering with the arguments for and against private healthcare. They might also actually compare them – "private healthcare is expensive but means you can access treatments, e.g. surgeries much faster, as the waiting lists are shorter. In private healthcare you can also request some treatments which you cannot do in the public system". This is not incorrect, but it does not address the question at hand.

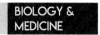

Q63: Should patients with a terminal illness be able to use an experimental drug, even if it has not yet been rigorously tested?

This is an ethical question: consider the 4 pillars of medical ethics – autonomy, justice, beneficence, non-maleficence. There is a lot more to say than these but this is a good way to get you started – make sure you evaluate each pillar properly in the context of the situation described in the question. Again, structure this answer with the pros and cons before coming to a conclusion. You must be able to defend your points.

Good applicant: Many issues are raised by this situation, and it is important to thoroughly assess the potential risks and benefits of experimental treatment. Looking at this using the 4 pillars of medical ethics can help. Respecting a patient's autonomy would involve a patient with the capacity to give informed consent (or not) to the treatment. The patient has to have capacity, meaning they can understand the information, weigh up pros and cons, make a decision and communicate that decision back. They must also be given all the information regarding the risky nature of the drug. There must be no pressure on the patient to choose either way or this undermines the principle of autonomy. Justice is the principle addressing the impact on the rest of society. On one hand, the drug may be very expensive and distributing it to one patient without an evidence base may divert resources from other treatments we know work. On the other hand, if the patient uses the drug as part of a clinical trial, it may advance our knowledge and enable wider access to the drug in the future. Conversely however, it may not be just to only use the sickest and most desperate patients as 'lab rats' for experimental drugs because they have no other choice.

Next is beneficence and non-maleficence. In this scenario the benefits and potential harms are not known as the drug is experimental. Every effort should be made to obtain knowledge on the toxicity/risks of the drug based on animal trials, similar drugs or modelling predictions. Furthermore, all other treatment avenues should be explored before settling on this high-risk option. However ultimately, I believe that it should be a decision made between treating clinician and an informed patient with capacity.

This answer provides a clear analysis of the four pillars and formulates a conclusion based on comments made previously.

A poor applicant may just address the issue as follows "a terminally ill patient might benefit from the drug as it could save their life or prolong it significantly, but it could also cause their last few months to be really painful and have a low quality of life. It is a risky decision that they would have to make." This answer does not say anything that is wrong but nor does it provide an answer that draws on ethical principles you should already know about. It also just states the obvious and doesn't provide any other insightful comments.

Q64: What is a clinical trial and why are they so important?

Clinical trials are the foundation of evidence-based medicine and whether you are interested in research or not you will find yourself involved in them somehow during your practicing life. This is a knowledge-based question – you should be able to comfortably define a clinical trial and explain how they function. Their importance is obvious and cannot be understated, but you should also be able to explain why this is the case. Bonus points if you can give examples of recent drugs or treatments approved – this shows interest in current healthcare news!

Good applicant: Clinical trials are medical research studies that look at the effect of an intervention on people. The intervention could be a drug, in which case it will have already been tested in the lab extensively before progressing to human trials, but it could also be surgical procedures or devices, screening tests and behavioural treatments. They aim to see if the treatment or procedure is safe, has any side effects, is beneficial compared to the current gold-standard treatment and its effect on quality of life. Clinical trials are prospective in nature and are usually randomised controlled trials.

There are 4 phases of clinical trials. Phase 1 aims to identify the safe dose range and any side effects in a small group of people, then phase 2 repeats the testing in a larger group of people to monitor adverse effects and then phase 3 looks at an even larger population and often compares the new treatment to the current gold standard treatment. Once the drug is approved for use in a country there will be a phase 4 trial which looks at the effect of the drug over a longer timeframe and may assess its cost-effectiveness as well.

They are vital for us to practice evidence-based medicine, meaning that we know our interventions will be useful for our patients. They allow us to quantify the risk vs benefits of interventions. Also, as clinical trials investigate which patient groups a treatment is most effective in, they are helpful to direct personalised medicine. Even if clinical trials show that the treatment doesn't work or that the side effects are too severe, the information is still useful for researchers and doctors and help direct future research. Without rigorous testing like clinical trials, drugs with unknown effects would be approved far more easily, and with no potential gain for patients. Patients would not be able to give informed consent to treatments if the clinicians themselves do not know enough about the drug. Clinical trials were very useful during the COVID-19 pandemic, as they showed the efficacy of drugs like dexamethasone and prevented any further gain of popularity of drugs like hydroxychloroquine.

A bad applicant would either define a clinical trial incorrectly or simply define it as being medical research trials in people but without delving any further into how they work nor what a good trial consists of. They would repeat the question by stating its importance, but without explaining anything. It's important to explain the use of clinical trials by highlighting their positive effects but also by explaining what would happen if they weren't in place.

Q65: Why are cancer cells more susceptible to destruction by radiotherapy than regular cells?

The question is straightforward and just knowledge-based – no real need for extra reading, just something that you should be able to extrapolate from A-level knowledge. Having said that, in the pressure of interview you might have a bit of a mind blank, or on the contrary, have a lot of ideas come to your mind – before you start answering take the time to think about what you want to say so that you can deliver a structured, logical and well-flowing answer as opposed to just 'knowledge dumping' everything you can think of.

A **good applicant**: Radiotherapy works by directing ionising radiation at cancerous cells which leads to DNA damage. Extensive DNA damage prevents cell division/replication and can induce cell death. Cancer cells are more radiosensitive because they are actively dividing (often following mutations in genes that control the cell cycle) and thus the impact of damaged DNA will be greater. Cells that are in the resting stage (G0) or divide less often, like most regular cells, are therefore less susceptible to the damage. The second thing that makes cancer cells more susceptible to destruction is that they often do not have intact DNA repair mechanisms. Tumours commonly have defects in the DNA repair genes as an initial mutation, which enables them to accumulate mutations in oncogenes or tumour-suppressor genes and propagate as a successful cancer. This means that when radiotherapy beams break the DNA or damage it even further, they have no means to repair it – in contrast to regular cells which can fix the DNA before the cell progresses any further in the cell cycle.

The answer addresses the question in a logical manner by first explaining how radiotherapy works and then with 2 clear points of why cancer cells are more susceptible.

A **poor applicant** might, as previously said, just knowledge dump on cancer and DNA but without communicating the reasons clearly and succinctly. They might also just have a limited understanding of the science behind it and say things that are incorrect.

Q66: If you had £1 billion to spend on a specific area of research, what would it be and why?

This question is attempting to see if the applicant has any knowledge of key research topics. It also is prompting them to discuss any particular areas of scientific interest that they have. What is most important with a question like this is the **justification** given for the area of research chosen. The interviewer could question why a certain area was chosen instead of another, but this is likely to get the interviewee to consider other options and back up their choice.

Good Applicant: If I had £1 billion to spend on any particular area of research, I would pick research into Alzheimer's disease. This is because it is a prevalent disease, primarily affecting older people. As there is an ageing population, it would be an advantageous area to research further in order to find a cure. At current, there are treatments that act to temporarily alleviate symptoms, but this does not prevent disease progression and the overall disease burden on both the patients, and their carers. The result of Alzheimer's disease, and therefore the symptoms of dementia, include a disturbance in cognitive functions including communication, memory, judgement amongst others. This can be particularly distressing for the patient, who may be very confused and agitated, as well as for the family, who may be primary carers. By funding research into Alzheimer's disease, treatments targeting amyloid plaque formation, for example, could be created. This is a potential avenue for treatment that could improve the lives of millions of people and reduce the stress of the disease on healthcare services, both in terms of support, and financially. If the research identified any environmental risk factors this could be used to inform the general public to make lifestyle changes or be implemented in a public health campaign to reduce the disease burden of Alzheimer's disease in the future. It could be a very beneficial research avenue, with the research money being used for large-scale trials in the cohort, imaging or for genetic sequencing, for example.

Poor Applicant: A poorer applicant might struggle to identify an area of research that they can justify investing such a large amount of money into or suggest a topic that perhaps would not need such money, for example a disease with a well-known cure. A poor candidate might change their mind when questioned on **why** a certain area of research was chosen. They may exhibit very limited knowledge of **how** we might go about researching a certain field and then implement that information through papers, peer review, publishing and campaigns.

Q67: What is the most significant medical breakthrough in the last 10 years?

This question is testing the applicant's knowledge of recent science, and current affairs. Medical schools will generally speaking be looking for you to be up-to-date on recent medical advances that have been in the news. Oxbridge, however, will be looking for a more scientific approach, likely based around papers/articles that you have read. <u>What</u> you choose is less important than how you justify it as the most significant breakthrough. Examples that could be used include: PrEP, CRISPR-Cas9 (more scientific), Ebola vaccine, COVID-19 vaccine

THE ULTIMATE OXBRIDGE INTERVIEW GUIDE: BIOLOGICAL SCIENCES **BIOLOGY & MEDICINE**

Good Applicant: I would say that the most significant medical breakthrough of the last 10 years is the advent of the PrEP medication now available to those at risk of HIV exposure. PrEP, unlike other HIV drugs, is for pre-exposure and therefore can prevent an individual from catching the virus in the first place. Following the HIV/AIDS epidemic in the 80s, which tore through many communities, drugs to slow the replication of the virus and prolong life began to be developed, for example, AZT. Anti-retroviral therapies became more widespread and a 'cocktail' of drugs became commonplace, in order to tackle the rapidly mutating HIV. Despite these treatments, nothing had yet been created that could protect those at risk from unknowingly acquiring the disease. PrEP has achieved this and provided another way to limit the spread of this virus. As a result of this, fewer people are contracting HIV, and consequentially fewer are developing AIDS. As well as reducing the incidence of the disease in those most at risk, the PrEP treatment has also had a knock-on effect, reducing the burden of AIDS-related diseases such as Kaposi's sarcoma on health services. All in all, it has saved many lives and is helping to limit the spread of this virus.

An answer such as the one above states the medical breakthrough, explains what it is and why it is helpful, and touches on the changes it can lead to in the future.

Poor Applicant: A poor answer would have little justification as to why this is a significant breakthrough, and may be lacking in the details, which could highlight a lack of background reading. The interviewer will be looking for scientific information as well as a personal 'weighing-up' of why this is important. Try to create a well-rounded answer.

Q68: What is an ECG and how does it work?

This question is focusing on the application of biological concepts in a clinical setting. Most applicants will know the general ideas of how blood flows through the heart as a result of the **myogenic** activity of pacemaker cells in the SAN. What will differentiate good and poor applicants is the extent of detail as to how the ECG represents this.

Good Applicant: An ECG is an **electrocardiogram**. This is a graph used in medical science that tracks the electrical activity of the heart, such that a trained eye can determine the heart rate and rhythms. A patient can be connected to the ECG via electrodes placed on their limbs and chest. Following this, a trace of the heart's electrical activity can be generated, as a result of depolarisation of the cardiac cells. Depolarisation is a change in polarity of the cell due to changes in ion distribution across the cell membrane. The electrical activity of the heart follows a specific pattern. First, an action potential is autogenerated by the sinoatrial node (the pacemaker of the heart) and spreads to the atria. The excitation spreads to the atrioventricular node, and via the bundle of His and Purkinje fibres to the apex of the heart. This then causes contraction from the bottom of the ventricles upwards, so that blood leaves the heart via the aorta and pulmonary arteries. This characteristic pattern of excitation gives rise to a characteristic ECG trace. This trace has key points such as the **P wave**, representing atrial depolarisation, the **QRS complex**, representing ventricular depolarisation and the **T wave** representing ventricular repolarisation. Using comparisons to the trace we'd expect from an ECG, a clinician can draw conclusions about a patient's cardiac activity and deduce if there are any conduction issues or rhythm changes, such as ventricular tachycardia. An ECG can form the basis of many diagnoses and be used to track the changes in a patient's condition.

Poor Applicant: A poor applicant might recognise what an ECG is to the extent of knowing that it is an electrocardiogram, and that it can provide an insight into the activity of the heart. They may, however, be lacking the scientific detail that the interviewer might be looking for. A lack of understanding of what each of the key points in our classical ECG trace represents might indicate gaps in core knowledge of cardiac activity. Most applicants will understand that it can play a key role in patient care and diagnosis but might be unable to name a specific example of a cardiac abnormality. All in all a poor applicant's answer will be lacking in detail.

Q69: How could you justify the legalisation of ecstasy?

This question considers the legal side of medicine, and how recreational drugs may cause a strain on medical resources. Drug legalisation is a controversial subject to some extent, as most illegal drugs will cause significant harm to patients if abused, but there are many arguments that decriminalisation will allow better regulation of their accessibility and reduce stigma whilst attempting to get help for any addiction issues.

Good Applicant: Legalisation of drugs, and in this case ecstasy, refers to the legal control of currently illegal drugs, in a similar way to how alcohol and tobacco are controlled. This approach would allow specific regulations to be put in place, to control access to and quality of these substances. At current, ecstasy could be seen as a 'gateway drug', and interaction with unregulated distributors could lead to exposure to other, more addictive substances. By legalising ecstasy, thus providing a safer, more controlled way to purchase it, there may be a removal of this exposure to 'harder' drugs. This, in turn, will benefit the individuals. Additionally, unregulated drug dealers may 'lace' drugs that they sell with even more harmful substances, putting the health of users at risk and adding to any strain on health services. By legalising ecstasy, quality of substances sold to those who want them can be checked, so that they know what they are consuming. All in all, legalising drugs may reduce strain on healthcare providers due to safer and more limited access. These substances could also be taxed to put back into public services, such as the NHS.

Furthermore, legalisation may reduce any shame around addiction issues, and assist people in asking for help, where before they may have felt nervous or scared of getting in trouble.

On the other hand, it could be argued that by making the usage of such addictive drugs more socially acceptable, people that otherwise wouldn't have been exposed will be encouraged to try them. This increase in usage in society could lead to more widespread drug abuse. Unfortunately, regulation does not prevent people from overdosing or becoming addicted, as we know from alcohol, and therefore more individuals may become dependent on legalised drugs such as ecstasy, harming themselves and increasing the burden on public health services. In order to justify the legalisation of ecstasy and similar drugs, in light of these arguments, perhaps certain limitations on the quantity you can purchase at any one time would have to be put in place. Additionally, more attention to and advertisement of services that help people with addiction, such that it doesn't become an endemic problem without a solution.

Poor Applicant: Most poor applicants will likely immediately say that no drugs should be decriminalised or legalised as they can be harmful, without proper consideration of the possible benefits. They might not weigh up both sides of the argument and as a result, form an unfounded conclusion based on bias. If they decide to attempt to justify the legalisation, their argument may lack a deeper explanation or perhaps exclude certain areas of the argument, such as controlling access to these drugs.

Q70: Should every hospital have an MRI machine?

This question aims to assess your ability to evaluate a given issue, make a balanced argument, consider all affecting factors and come to a valid conclusion. MRI scanners are an extremely useful tool in medicine. They are often considered to be the gold standard for diagnosing brain tumours and used to detect other conditions like osteomyelitis (infection of the bone). MRIs can form detailed images, but also have several drawbacks. You might want to think about the reasons why, if MRI scanners are so useful, there are hospitals that presently don't have one. This would include factors like cost or an alternative device that is used instead. If you do mention alternatives, you should explore why they are considered to be a better option to MRIs.

A **good candidate** could say, *"MRI scanners are machines that can be used to view internal tissues and body structures and I am aware that they are commonly used to diagnose tumours. They have many advantages over other forms of imaging as they do not expose the patient to radiation and are able to provide images of soft tissue within the body at a higher resolution than most other imaging can. However, I know that they also have several disadvantages. As they create an image using magnetic fields, the scanners cannot be used for patients with pacemakers or metal replacements. Many people may also feel claustrophobic in the machine as it surrounds their whole body and creates a lot of noise, unlike a CT scanner. However, I think that the biggest reason that all hospitals cannot have an MRI scanner is because they are extremely expensive to both buy and use. Even though I know that MRIs are more detailed in their images, I feel that the funds saved by using alternatives such a CT can be used to pay for treatments where there aren't alternatives available, e.g., a new life-saving cancer drug. Moreover, a doctor who believes that a patient is in real need of an MRI scan can still refer them to another hospital for the scan, despite the inconvenience. Whereas, an understaffed ward can prove fatal for the patients on it, if the NHS doesn't have the budget to employ enough doctors per shift. In an ideal world, every hospital would have an MRI scanner but the reality is, with the budget the NHS operates under, I feel that alternatives such as CT scanners would be a better use of funds."*

There is no right answer here, but the conclusion that you come to must be sufficiently backed up by a set of logical reasons. When you name a factor, you must fully explain why it is relevant to your conclusion. They want to be able to see how you came to a decision, and for you to justify your rationale.

For example, a **poor candidate** may answer with *"No, because MRI machines are expensive"*. Like the good candidate, they have also identified cost as a factor. However, without explaining the implications of these machines having such a high cost (if every hospital were to have one), they have not displayed the evaluation and decision-making skills that the interviewer is looking for. The same goes for giving points for only one side of the argument. They are looking for you to assess both the benefits and drawbacks, so as to arrive at a well-thought-out, carefully considered conclusion.

Q71: What are the ethical implications of genetic screening in utero?

Ethics questions are common at interview – their purpose is to allow the interviewers to assess your morals and integrity. Probity is a value that is outlined in the GMC guidelines and is an essential quality to have a doctor.

Always define the question in your introduction to show you understand what they are asking, especially if they are using specialised terminology like 'genetic screening'. This question is an ethical scenario, so you can answer it using the 4 pillars of medical ethics, i.e., autonomy, beneficence, non-maleficence and justice. You should know what each of these terms means and be able to apply them to medical dilemmas. When answering questions like these, start your argument with the ethical pillar that you think is most relevant and then work through all 4 of them in order of significance to the question.

A **good candidate** may respond with, *"Genetic screening involves testing individuals to determine whether or not they have a genetic condition. During pregnancy, women whose children are at risk of inheriting a genetic disease, like cystic fibrosis, or developing a chromosomal condition, like Down's syndrome, may be offered genetic screening in utero to check whether their child has any such condition. If testing shows that the foetus is positive for a genetic disease, the parents may consider having an abortion. Abortion is the termination of a pregnancy resulting in the death of the embryo or foetus. This is an ethical dilemma and can therefore be approached using the 4 pillars of medical ethics. Under the pillar autonomy, it is the choice of the pregnant woman what happens to her body. There are people who argue that the foetus should have a right to 'decide' as well and therefore believe that abortion should not be allowed. But currently, the woman has autonomy over her body and can choose to abort the foetus up to 24 weeks. For beneficence, as an adult the foetus would likely view the abortion not being carried out in as a good thing. Under non-maleficence, you would be terminating a pregnancy and therefore directly killing the foetus. On the other hand, the mother may experience psychological trauma or emotional harm if they would like to abort their child and the abortion is not allowed to occur. Furthermore, going through with the abortion may reduce the suffering that the foetus would have to endure due to their genetic condition later in life. Finally under justice, if the genetic condition that the foetus has requires consistent medical help and frequent hospitalisations, the abortion could save valuable resources which may be allocated to treat someone else. These are the main factors to be considered when debating the ethical implications of genetic screening."*

You must not express your personal bias, if you have one, and let it affect your answer. They want you to be able to tackle the question from an objective point of view. A **poor candidate** could say, *"Genetic screening is unethical as it could result in an abortion, this is against my beliefs."* This would reflect the candidate's individual prejudice, rather than having them gauge the dilemma from a neutral perspective and present a fair argument.

Q72: Should placebos be used in hospitals? What about GP surgeries?

You should begin by defining the term 'placebo' and explaining the benefits of the placebo effect (the phenomenon that can be caused by taking a placebo). You need to identify that using the placebo effect to treat patients, in both hospitals and GP surgeries, would involve lying to the patient and you must explore the consequences of this.

Good candidate's response: *"A placebo is a substance that has no therapeutic effect, but looks like and is presented to the patient taking it as a 'real drug'. Sometimes taking such a substance can lead to the 'placebo effect', where an individual may feel better or experience some sort of benefit from taking the substance, which cannot be attributed to its properties. This is a psychological phenomenon, but can still cause the patient to experience real improvements in their physical or mental health. However, for the placebo effect to work, a patient must believe that they are taking a real and effective drug, rather than the 'fake' placebo. This would require a doctor to lie to their patients about the medication that they are being prescribed, which is unethical. It undermines the trust that a patient may have in their doctor and could severely damage their doctor-patient relationship. If the patient were to realise that the drug they are taking is a placebo, they may feel stupid or betrayed, which could make them hesitant to seek medical help from their doctor in the future. It is also important to maintain that trust between doctors and patients, because it is only when patients trust and feel safe with their doctor in all respects, that they will be willing and comfortable discussing potentially embarrassing problems that they have been experiencing with their health. Using placebos to treat patients, in both hospitals and GP surgeries, could also cause them severe medical harm in certain situations. If the patient happens to visit a different doctor who is unaware of their situation, they may incorrectly state to the doctor that they are on a certain medication, rather than a placebo. This could cause the doctor to prescribe the patient a different course of treatment based on this false information, rather than the course of treatment that would be best for them. It could be argued that using placebos may save a lot of time and money.*

For example, individuals with Munchausen syndrome could be dealt with more easily by prescribing them a cheap placebo, so that expensive resources and valuable time is not wasted treating an individual with a supposedly fake illness, who repeatedly insists that they are sick. Furthermore, people who experience a real benefit from the placebo effect would avoid experiencing any of the nasty side effects that a real drug may have. Still, I think that the harm that could be caused by using placebos to treat patients, much outweighs any of the benefits they provide. Therefore, no placebos should not be used in hospitals or GP surgeries."

Poor candidate's response: *"Placebos should be used to treat patients, because lying to a patient is okay if it is going to save time and money"*. This goes without saying, but you should never promote any behaviour that is clearly unethical in your answers, especially when there is an obvious alternative solution available. They want to see someone who will be honest and practice ethical medicine in the future.

Q73: How would you differentiate between salt and sugar without tasting them?

The interviewers have asked you this question to test your problem-solving skills. Additionally, they'd like to see how you handle a question where the obvious answer is not an option. They want you to think about the question scientifically, thus eliminating the most clear-cut answer, i.e., tasting the 2 substances, to push you in that direction.

There are a few different ways you can choose to answer this question. Having said that, they all come down to the same basics – bonding and structure. From GCSE Chemistry, you should know that the chemical formula of salt is $NaCl$, which is an ionic compound. Similarly, from first year A-level Biology you should be aware that sucrose is a disaccharide, formed from 2 monosaccharide sugar molecules joined by a glyosidic bond. You can infer that it is, thus, roughly twice the size of 1 molecule of glucose and you know that it is a covalent compound. Now that you can deduce the chemical properties of the 2 compounds from their formulae, you could theoretically use their differences to distinguish between them.

For example, you can identify each compound by testing their electrical conductivity in a solution, determining their boiling points or dissolving each substance in alcohol. If you have time, you could mention all 3 methods, but describing just 1 is sufficient. When answering this question, make sure you fully explain your thought process.

Good candidates may reply with, "I know that salt, or NaCl, is an ionic compound and that sugar, or sucrose, is covalent. Therefore, if I were to dissolve both substances in water, making up 2 separate solutions, only the salt solution would have the capacity to conduct electricity. So, to distinguish between the solutions I would set up 2 simple circuits, consisting of a small lightbulb, cell and wires and incorporate each solution into a different circuit. The circuit whose light bulb subsequently starts glowing is the circuit that contains the salt solution rather than the sugar one.

A **poor candidate** may simply say they "don't know" or mention a trivial difference like, "salt and sugar look different." If you can't come up with an answer straight away, do not worry about it. The interviewers are there to help out and will prompt you if necessary.

Q74: What do you understand by the words perception, self-awareness and consciousness?

This question may seem bizarre for a medical interview. Its purpose could be to test your clarity of thought. This is your ability to take one of your ideas, package it up and present it to the interviewers neatly, concisely, and understandably. This is a vital skill for decision-making. You should define each of the expressions in your own words and if you have time, explain how they relate to medicine.

Good candidate's response: "My understanding of perception is that is it an individual's point of view or image of a person, event or object based on the set of their experiences that relate to that thing. For instance, someone's perception of an individual would depend upon either the interactions that they'd had with that person or the things they had heard about them. When reading an autobiography, you develop an image of the person that you are reading about. I would call that your perception of them. Self-awareness involves someone's unbiased perception of themselves. It is being aware of your own lifestyle, routine and actions. A person who is self-aware realises their own strengths and shortcomings. Finally, consciousness is to recognise and process something. To be conscious of something is to be aware of it. Perception, self-awareness and consciousness are necessary skills for doctors. They must be perceptive of changes in their patients' health or behaviour that could be a result of an underlying medical cause. Doctors should be conscious of their patient's situation, this is not limited to their physical health but also their mental wellbeing. This is important in trying to practice holistic medicine, where you are treating a person and not just the disease. It builds the doctor-patient relationship so that patients can trust and feel comfortable with their doctors. It is only then that they will be willing to disclose potentially embarrassing problems that they have been facing with their health. Doctors can only treat these problems effectively if they know about them and have all the information. Self-awareness allows doctors to learn from their mistakes and improve to provide better care for future patients."

Poor candidate's response would be to panic. When you get asked a weird question like this, don't panic. Take a minute to collect your thoughts and understand the question. When you are ready to answer, structure it so that it is clear detailed and thorough. It is much better if you wait and come out with a succinct and full answer, than if you reply immediately but scatter your thoughts. The interviewers will appreciate if you take the time to think but then come out with a crisp response.

Q75: How many litres of blood does your heart pump in your lifetime?

This is a classic Oxbridge question in the sense that they are notorious for asking questions that may seem impossible at first, but are actually relatively simple to work out. Do not worry if your final answer is incorrect. They care more about your method than the exact accuracy of the number you end up with. The most important advice here is to 'think out loud'. They want to witness your critical thinking skills in action. Furthermore, don't be afraid to ask for extra information if you find that you don't have everything needed for your calculation.

A **good candidate** will say, "I'm aware that the average person's heart rate when at rest is 80 beats per minute. Although a person's heart rate would not stay constant at this rate throughout their entire life (e.g., their heart rate would increase during exercise), I will still use 80 bpm for my calculation to keep things simple. I am not quite sure what the average person's stroke volume would be, am I allowed to ask you this?" *The interviewers tell you that the average stroke volume for an adult is 50 ml* "Using the formula cardiac output = stroke volume × heart rate, I now know that every minute the average adult human heart pumps 50 × 80 = 4000 ml of blood. I'm going to assume that the average person's life span is 80 years, so there are 80 × 365 × 24 × 60 = 42,048,000 (Ask for a calculator at this point!) minutes in a person's lifetime. It is worth noting that before an individual reaches adulthood, their stroke volume is likely to be less than 50 ml as they are not fully grown. For the sake of convenience, I am going to ignore this. In conclusion, this means that in total a human heart pumps 4000 × 42048000 = 1.68192×10^{11} ml or 1.68192×10^{8} litres in its lifetime."

A **poor candidate** may just blurt out a number without discussing their approach to the question. This is useless to the interviewers, who are trying to evaluate your problem-solving capabilities. Make sure that you take them through each step of your working to explain how you arrived at your solution.

Q76: Why do the atria contract before the ventricles?

This question aims to give the interviewers an opportunity to examine your analytical skills. You need to contemplate the different possible models for the cardiac cycle and start to eliminate each of them by explaining why they can't occur. Using this process, you will find that there is only 1 suitable model – which basically is the point of this question. This will reveal the reasons for which the atria contract before the ventricles and will therefore lead you to your answer.

Good candidate's response: "The function of the atria is to receive blood from their respective blood vessels and then contract so that this blood flows into the ventricles. Suppose we consider what would happen if the atria didn't contract before the ventricles. There are only 2 other possibilities: either the atria contract after the ventricles, or the atria and ventricles contract at the same time. If the atria were to contract after the ventricles, there would be no blood in the ventricles to pump out of the heart. This would defeat the purpose of the cardiac cycle and render the heart useless. If the atria and ventricles were to contract at the same time, blood would not be able to move into the ventricles as there would be high pressure and no space in the ventricle cavities. This may even result in the back flow of blood back into atria and then the vena cava and pulmonary vein. I can imagine this could also significantly damage the heart valves. Therefore, the only feasible model is for the atria of the heart to contract before the ventricles."

A **poor candidate** may say, "because the heart is designed that way." This is obvious. They want you to figure out why it is designed that way. Make it apparent that you can think quickly on the spot in a logical but coherent manner. Sometimes your answer may not be completely correct but as long as it is plausible and makes sense, the interviewers will be satisfied with it.

Q77: Why do we need ATP? Why not just release energy from glucose directly?

The purpose of this question is to allow you to demonstrate your ability to reason your way through a problem. Having studied the first year of A-level Biology, you will know that ATP is a relatively small molecule compared to glucose. What is the significance of this? To figure out the solution, think about the role of ATP and what would happen if it were to be substituted with glucose.

Good candidate's response: "I know that each glucose molecule produces 30-40 molecules of ATP via aerobic respiration. I imagine that means that glucose is far larger than ATP and thus also holds much more energy in its bonds. If glucose were to be used as the 'currency' for energy in the body instead of ATP, massive amounts of energy would have to be released at a single location. This could cause a lot of damage and possibly denature essential enzymes in the cell. It would also be very inefficient as there would be surplus energy wasted for each process that doesn't require the full volume of energy provided by a single glucose molecule. ATP provides energy in small packets and can also be broken down in a single step, this makes it a much better energy 'currency' than glucose."

Poor Candidate's response: "You probably could release energy directly from glucose, but that's just not the way it works." Firstly, this answer is incorrect. The candidate has given absolutely no thought to the question and has not even bothered to justify their response. The interviewers have asked you this question for a reason. There is only 20-30 minutes per interview so they will not waste time on a question that doesn't tell them anything. Most Oxbridge interview questions will target your problem-solving skills so if the answer isn't obvious at first, try to think outside the box. The questions are made to be slightly obscure so that they make you think as the interviewers want to see that you can work through to suggest a solution.

Q78: What is DNA fingerprinting and why is it used in forensics?

This question is assessing both your A-level biology knowledge and your ability to think critically. Everyone's DNA is unique, except for twins who are genetically identical. Think about how this makes DNA fingerprinting so useful, especially in a forensic setting.

Good candidate's response: "DNA fingerprinting is a method used to produce a specific pattern of DNA bands from an individual's genome. Each person's DNA is unique so the pattern produced by their genome is specific to that person. This means that if the DNA profile of a sample found at a crime matched the DNA sample of a potential suspect, that individual must have been at that location at some point in recent history. This can be used to place suspects at a crime scene or put a weapon in their hands. For example, if a murder were to occur where a person was stabbed to death, while holding the knife the killer may accidently cut themselves and draw blood. If the weapon were to be found, DNA fingerprinting could be used to confirm that there are 2 people's blood on the weapon with only one matching the victim's DNA. It can presumed that the other person whose blood is present is the killer and again their identity could be confirmed using DNA fingerprinting. As DNA profiles are specific to individuals, it is a certainty that the suspect has held the knife before. Combined with other evidence, the killer can be caught and proved guilty using this technique."

Poor candidate's response: "Fingerprinting is the process of using the pattern's on a person's finger to identify them, etc." The candidate has misunderstood the question and is thus answering incorrectly. It's easy to get confused with similar sounding terminology at interview, especially if you're nervous. That's why it is important to listen carefully to the question being asked and make sure you understand it. If you aren't quite sure what the interviewers are getting at, ask for clarification because they can word the same question slightly differently to help you.

Q79: Has the enhancement of medical knowledge destroyed human evolution?

Questions like these are designed to stimulate curiosity and provoke discussion. This topic is slightly controversial so it is an opportunity for them to probe you about your thinking. There is no right answer here. Engage with their comments but also fight your corner. They may try to put you off but do not give in, if they are clearly being belligerent, they may be trying to see if you can uphold your own argument under pressure. As long as your response is logical and well-reasoned, you're doing good.

A **good candidate** could say, "I'd argue that it is civilisation rather than the enhancement of medical knowledge that has destroyed human evolution. An inherited disease would only be affected by natural selection, and eventually removed from the gene pool, if it caused the individual or either die before they produce offspring or to become infertile. In the wild, adaptations such as long legs, which could help you run faster, would be selected for as they would help humans evade their predators or catch more prey and this be more likely to survive to childbearing age. Inherited diseases that we treat today like sickle cell anaemia and Huntington's disease do not kill a person before they can have children, so extending their life beyond childbearing through the enhancement of medical knowledge would not influence evolution and indeed genetic screening could prevent these genes from being passed on. As far as I can think right now, there are very few inherited diseases that have an early enough onset such that the individual does not have offspring and cannot pass the gene on. The only example of a disease I can think of like this is Type I diabetes mellitus which can start in childhood. We now use insulin to treat this, but before its discovery I suppose that children diagnosed with T1DM would die young. This would lead to natural selection as affected individuals may not produce offspring and thus the faulty allele would become less prevalent in the gene pool over time. In this case, the enhancement of medical knowledge has destroyed evolution as patients with diabetes can now be treated and lead a relatively normal life, which includes having children and passing their genes on. Therefore, I'd like to change my answer and say yes, in some cases the enhancement of medical knowledge has destroyed evolution.

A **poor candidate** may answer, "Yes, the enhancement of medical knowledge has destroyed evolution because people are now living longer." There are many things wrong here. The statement is very general and the candidate has not explained why living longer would affect human evolution. They also haven't specified that living longer only influences evolution if it means that an organism that would have otherwise died before having children, then lives long enough to pass on their genes to their offspring. If the candidate had gone into more detail with their response, they may have realised this and been able to correct themselves. It is crucial in Oxbridge interviews to always explain your answers fully and justify any of your reasons. They are looking for students they will potentially be teaching next year so you need to portray yourself as someone who they would want to teach, i.e. be intellectually curious and think critically.

Q80: Why are infectious diseases no longer the biggest killer in the UK?

This question is somewhat topical in nature. You should know from extra reading what the biggest killers in the UK are, but you may not know why they are more deadly per se than infectious diseases. Notice the question says that infectious diseases are 'no longer' the biggest killer – this implies that they once were. Consider what has changed over the past few decades that could have prevented so many people dying from infectious diseases. Remember to explicate your thinking.

Good candidate's response: "Previously deadly infectious diseases can now be easily treated using modern medicine. For instance, the Black Death, one of the deadliest pandemics in history, was caused by the bacterium *Yersinia pestis*, which could now be cured by using antibiotics. This goes for the majority of bacterial infections now that would have otherwise killed people in the past. Viruses are other infectious agents that have been well controlled in recent decades. Vaccines have been developed to combat viruses, e.g., the viral disease smallpox was eradicated using a vaccine. Furthermore, education about the transmission of such infectious diseases has become more widespread. Awareness about the precautions that can be taken to prevent transmission may have also played a major role in reducing the deaths caused by infectious diseases. People are now aware that HIV and Hepatitis C are blood-borne diseases that can be sexually transmitted so the use of protection is encouraged and screening of donor blood before blood transfusions has become common practice. All this means that ultimately less people die from infectious diseases and deaths from conditions like heart-attacks and strokes that are more spontaneous or from late-stage cancers that are difficult to detect become a more common cause. Surprisingly, dementia is the number one killer in the UK. This may be because people are living longer so diseases associated with old age are becoming more prevalent. People are also most likely to succumb to these diseases, like Alzheimer's disease, because we do not have cures for them yet."

Poor candidate's response: "Heart-attacks are more deadly than most infectious diseases so infectious diseases cannot be the biggest killer in the UK." The problem with this answer is that the candidate has not explained why heart-attacks are more deadly than infectious diseases in today's world. They have not addressed the fact that infectious diseases were once the biggest killer in the UK or explored that steps have been taken over the years to reduce the number of deaths that they cause. The question asks you to explain the reasons why infectious diseases are not the biggest killer in the UK anymore, which the candidate has not done.

Q81: Would it matter if tigers became extinct?

This question is reflective of the kind of question which you should be asking yourself when you're answering a number of the other questions in this book, particularly those about which factor is most important out of a range of options. It can seem as though there is no answer to 'would it matter?' questions which doesn't rely on your own internal gut instinct. However, you should still try to justify your reasoning as far as possible, or state where you are making leaps based on 'gut instinct' (as it isn't inherently a bad thing).

A **poor answer** may be something like the following:

"Of course it would, changing even small factors in the environment has a big impact, so changing something as significant as whether there is a predator at the top of certain food chains would make a massive difference".

Or, the following:

"Not really, ecosystems are generally pretty adaptable, and things have gone extinct before".

Both of these are weak answers because they don't start by considering what we mean when we ask if something 'matters'. While the long-term effects might be part of how we decide if it 'matters' it isn't the only factor.

A **good answer** would therefore begin by considering a range of reasons why it might or might not matter, before coming to a judgement. These reasons might include:

- What would the short and long term effects on the environment be?
- What would the short and long term effects on other animals be?
- Is there an inherent value to biodiversity?
- When an animal (any animal) becomes extinct, is the loss of knowledge or loss of potential significant?

The **best answers** would be able to bring together a consideration of all of the above factors, before giving a single judgement on whether it would matter or not. Importantly, it would show a nuanced consideration of what the statement 'this does matter' or 'this doesn't matter' means. If we say 'it wouldn't matter' does that inherently mean that we wouldn't or shouldn't care or try to prevent it? If we say it does matter – are there limits on how much we would actually do anything about that?

Q82: Why do cats' eyes appear to 'glow' in the dark?

Although it may seem like there is a single correct answer to this question, it is possible to give a very good interview answer without knowing anything about the science behind the solution before you begin. And similarly, it's perfectly possible to know the answer before you start and give a very poor reasoning – so be careful.

A **poor answer** would generally be quite limited and vague, something like:

"They're probably made of a different sort of material or cell which glows in the dark".

The problem that the candidate is having here, is that they're assuming that this is an answer that they can't break down – either they know it or they don't. As a result, they're limited in what they feel they can say because they're missing this knowledge. This isn't true.

A **good answer** would start by explaining what is going on for the eyes to 'glow'. For example,

"If they're glowing in the dark, that means that there is light which is originally in the cats eye, which is being reflected back outwards which we then see".

This forms an excellent starting point, as it poses a number of questions which the student can then explore (either independently, or when prompted by their interviewer). For example, what might be causing the reflection? Is the reflection intentional? What would be the benefit to the cat (if any) of this reflection?

The **best answers** would work logically through these questions, working in discussion with the interviewer, and based on the starting point above, to develop an answer such as the following:

"Given cats are nocturnal, it seems as though their eyes would be adapted to work in very low light conditions, and so its quite odd that they'd be reflecting light back out of their eye"

"I don't think that the glow would be an intentional feature, at least, I can't currently think of a reason that would benefit them. Perhaps they are reflecting the light for a different reason, and some of it accidentally escapes back out through their pupil."

"Yes, I think that maybe they're reflecting the light to try and get as much of the light to hit their retina as possible, even if it didn't hit the retina initially, and some of it must be reflected back out by accident"

Follow up questions might explore whether this is something that happens in all animals, how it happens (by material/shape/design of the eye), etc…

Q83: What do you think the impact of epigenetic research is on medical treatment?

This question relies on you having at least a passing understanding of what is meant by 'epigenetics' before you start. If this is something that you have researched, or read about during your preparation, then you should start by explaining what you understand it to mean, so that you give the interviewers an opportunity to clarify or correct any areas which they understand differently before you begin. If you don't know what is meant by epigenetics, the interviewers may give you a prompt such as:

"Epigenetics is the study of heritable changes to an organisms characteristics which aren't related to changes to the genetic code, but rather are in addition to the genetic code and influence the way such code is expressed".

A **poor answer** would struggle to link epigenetics to medical treatment, or show an understanding of what is meant by epigenetics on even a simple level.

A **good answer** might start by giving some examples of epigenetic changes which could be observed in people. For example, there is a large area of study related to examining whether there are epigenetic markers in the offspring of Holocaust survivors which lead to the increased susceptibility to stress, anxiety and other mental health conditions in this group. They would then go onto to examine whether this additional form of inheritance would impact medical treatment, for example by encouraging pre-emptive treatment in groups which may show this susceptibility without the need for genetic testing or manifestation of the disorder.

The **best answers** might go one step further, in order to consider the effect of epigenetics on research into new treatments. For example, if it was found to be easier (or more ethically acceptable) to influence epigenetic inheritance than changing people's genetic code itself, could this be used to influence gene expression without the need for less acceptable genetic modification of people.

Q84: Do you think the NHS should advocate vegetarianism or veganism as a means to combat public health issues with obesity?

Questions about public health policy are not uncommon in medical interviews, at Oxbridge and other universities. This is because policies for social prescribing, and government-led initiatives for maintaining public health are often considered very separately to typical healthcare decisions. However, they are clearly intricately linked, and as a future doctor, will be something that you interact with in your patients on a regular basis.

A **poor answer** may give an imbalanced answer, which focussed solely on the positives or negatives of vegan and vegetarian diets. Alternatively the candidate may speak convincingly about both the pros and cons of vegan and vegetarian diets for individuals, but fail to link this to whether the NHS should be publicly supporting these diets, and the impact this would have on public health. It is important to remember that the question being asked here isn't about whether any single individual should adopt a particular diet to combat their individual health conditions. The question is seeking to examine your understanding of the role of the state-funded health service, how public health campaigns work, and the ethical issues surrounding both.

A **good answer** would, in general, begin by accepting the premise that vegetarian diets could reduce obesity, and then examine whether it is ethical for the NHS to be advocating for them. Given the challenges of being a vegetarian or vegan for many people, which include personal preferences as well as cost, difficulty finding ingredients or time to cook, the candidate should explore whether this would be as effective as a marketing approach as other campaigns such as the '5 a day' or 'Couch to 5k' or 'Change for Life' campaigns which have all been seen recently.

The **best answers** would show a clear understanding that this is, first and foremost, a question of numbers. How many people would be receptive to this messaging? What would be the impact of this messaging on those people? Would smaller changes in a larger proportion of the population bring about a greater benefit to the public *on average*, and simultaneously reduce cost to the NHS?

Q85: How do stem cells become specialised?

This question is asking about a topic which will have been studied by the majority of students multiple times by the time they reach their Oxbridge interview – stem cell specialisation. It is important to note that it's not asking you to describe stem cell specialisation, explain what cells stem cells can specialise into, or even discuss the ethical issues surrounding stem cell research, all of which are more common in GCSE and A-level specifications. Instead, it is asking about the way in which the stem cells become specialised – how do they know what to specialise into? What triggers the process of specialisation?

A **poor candidate** might approach this question by simply listing everything they know about stem cells based on their academic study:

"Stem cells are undifferentiated... found in bone marrow... adult stem cells can only become one of a small number of specialised cells... embryonic stem cells can differentiate more... there are ethical issues due to the use of stem cells in medical research".

While none of this is incorrect, it also fails to address the question, and so wouldn't be a good answer to this question at interview.

A **good candidate** might briefly summarise the information above, before beginning to consider situations in which stem cells need to become specialised. Although this won't directly answer the question, it might give hints to allow the candidate to be able to deduce how the process works.

They then might go onto discuss what inhibits the ability of cells to become other specialised cells. If each of your cells contains your genetic information, why are some cells restricted to express certain genes and other cells others? By considering whether specialisation is a default state which is inhibited, or is an unusual state, the candidate might be able to propose ways in which specialisation could be triggered.

Q86: The Pernkopf Topographic Anatomy of Man is often regarded as the most comprehensive book of human anatomy in the world and is of immeasurable use to surgeons and other medical professionals as a result. It was also developed through human experimentation under the Nazis. Should we stop using or publishing it?

This question is one of many which could focus on the history of medicine and medical research, which is often grey and at times categorically unethical. The result of this challenging history in the field is that much of our understanding of human physiology today is based on unethical, non-consensual research, largely conducted against minority groups. The question therefore boils down to a question of whether the continued use of research which was conducted in such an unethical manner implies tacit acceptance. And alternatively, whether the reduction of knowledge or resources which would result from the removal of the research which came from these unethical foundations could itself be an ethical problem, given the harm which may arise to people being treated now.

A **poor answer** would fail to show an appreciation of the fact this is a grey area which is widely discussed and revisited in the profession. It isn't simply an exercise for an interview. As a result answers such as these, lack the nuance of a successful answer:

"No, we shouldn't stop using it. The people affected by the research won't be less affected if we stop, so it would be completely pointless and just hurt people now."

"Yes, we absolutely should stop using it. There's no justification for continuing to use resources which we know were created unethically, except to show that the medical profession doesn't really have a problem with what happened after all".

Neither of these show any consideration of the other side of the 'argument', and as a result close down any possibility of discussion with the interviewer.

A **good answer** would consider arguments for and against the continued use of such books, before coming to their own conclusion.

The **best answers** would link their reasoning to pillars of medical ethics, as well as potentially incorporating ethical frameworks (such as a utilitarian approach or virtue ethics) which they could use to make their decision.

In this case, it is worth noting that while the book is still widely in use it has not been published for some time.

Q87: What is a neurotransmitter?

Any knowledge you have on neurotransmitters prior to your interview will definitely help with this question, however, you should be able to work out some key points even if you were unfamiliar.

A **poor answer** might be unfamiliar and unable to work out what a neurotransmitter is, even with prompting from the interviewer. If you didn't know what a neurotransmitter was, even a statement such as this one would be a good start, to allow the interviewer to then introduce the concept further: *"The neuro- bit tells me it's something that occurs in your brain, and it's transmitting something in your brain. So I'd guess it's something that either transfers signals in your brain, or material like blood or hormones, perhaps".*

A **good answer** would ensure the use of specific language in its description (e.g. synapses, neuron, chemical markers) as much as possible. It may also include the sketching of a diagram to explain where the neurotransmitter would be found, and why it is important (why can't neurons just join up end-to-end-to-end endlessly?). Importantly, neurotransmitters aren't solely found between neurons (an error made by many candidates), but can also be found at any point in the receptor-effector pathway for example, between neurons and muscle cells or gland cells depending on the pathway being discussed.

The **best answers** may include examples of neurotransmitters which the candidate was familiar with (such as dopamine or serotonin). This would then allow the candidate to build on their knowledge about the role of dopamine and serotonin in the brain, to give a more generalised explanation of the wider processes in the brain which neurotransmitters contribute to.

Further questions could then be asked by the interviewer about ways in which neurons or neurotransmitters could 'malfunction', the consequences if they did, and the ways in which this might be targeted by treatment.

Q88: What are QALYs?

As with several of the other questions discussed previously it's important to understand what the question is actually asking you to talk about before you answer.

A **very poor candidate** may not have heard of QALYs. Although in general, you aren't expected to be an expert before the interview (otherwise, why would you need to study?!), you are expected to have demonstrated an interest in and understanding of the state of the profession in the UK. Understanding issues such as resource distribution decisions by NICE, and the ethical quandaries which surround those decisions is a significant part of this.

A **poor candidate** will simply define QALYs as 'Quality-adjusted life years'.

An **average candidate** may build on this to attempt to explain what that definition means. Perhaps explaining that a quality-adjusted life year is the equivalent number of years of perfect health which a person has. So for a person with a very low quality of life, although they may be expected to live another 50 years, their QALYs may be a much smaller value (e.g. 1 or 2) when their illness is taken into account.

Even this average candidate is somewhat missing the point of the question. The interviewers know what QALYs are, and aren't seeking to test your knowledge – because they're intending to teach you quite a bit more once you join the university! So what is the point of the question?

An **excellent candidate** would attempt to explain what QALYs seek to achieve, and by extension, why they exist, and what their place is in the medical profession. For example, following the explanation above, they may go on to say something like 'QALYs are an attempt to quantify a value for the remaining years of a patient's life, in order to allow comparisons to be made between people with vastly different life expectancies and health issues'. And this is getting to the heart of the question. QALYs are, fundamentally, a blunt instrument which is used to simplify the vast spectrum of human health and experience down to a single value which can then be used to justify treatment options and expense.

This then leads to a discussion about how QALYs are calculated, the ethics behind the decisions which are made, and the difficulties of withholding treatment in favour of other patients in certain cases. Importantly, the very best candidates will be able to acknowledge both the ethical issues, their personal viewpoint, and the reality of the situation in their answer. It may be that you personally find the whole idea of QALYs ethically dubious (you would not be alone in that!), and it wouldn't be wrong to give this as an opinion at interview, as long as you could also temper this with your understanding of the necessity behind why they exist.

Many things in modern medicine, and in particular in public health, are based on a least-worst option – and your understanding of this, alongside how you would relate to it as a medical student and doctor is what's really being tested here.

Q89: Why can you stay balanced whilst cycling, but not on a stationary bike?

Although many medical students won't have studied physics formally since GCSE, it is worth brushing up on some of the fundamentals. Many medical students don't realise how much physics can be found in some of their upcoming lectures (biomechanical modelling of joints, for example, draws heavily from physics ideas relating to resolving forces and relating force to extension and compression of materials). As a result, this question aims to be a taster of the kind of 'scientific common sense' which you may have to use in during your time at medical school (and beyond).

A **poor answer** will normally incorrectly identify the source of the balance issues, as a quirk of human anatomy, and often (given the question asks about balance) incorrectly identify the ear as the culprit. This leads to a situation of trying to justify why your inner ear would be incapable of balancing unless you're moving forward, which is unlikely to be successful.

A **good answer** will normally start with a diagram – what are the forces on you, the cyclist, while you're in motion? How do these forces differ if you're stationary? From this, you can pull out some conclusions about what might be affecting the ability to balance. Some students may mention that the momentum of the bike means you'll continue moving forward even if you begin to wobble – but may not fully be able to expand on why this would make balance easier.

The **best answers** will identify that balance when the bike is stationary is based on constant tiny adjustments to your position. They may be familiar with the concept of angular momentum, or at least able to draw analogies to other situations in which objects have a tendency to stay upright only if they're moving (for example, spinning tops). Drawing these comparisons, or related examples will then help you to consider which muscles you would need to use to stay upright. Similarly, unicyclists can stay upright, but have greater difficulty and need to make more adjustments using their own strength – a consideration of the differences may help you to structure an answer here.

Q90: Why are BAME people more likely to die of covid than the general population?

Questions about the covid-19 pandemic, its causes, effects, and the response, are all highly likely to arise in interviews for some considerable time. As a result, it is worth looking beyond generic media examination of the pandemic (of which there is more than you could hope to read in preparation for your interview) and focus on the response of organisations representing medical professionals, for example, SAGE, the 'alternative SAGE', or the BMJ.

This question is asking about a highly relevant area of discussion within medicine, with research showing worse outcomes for minority groups undergoing a range of different treatments (not just for covid). This often appears to remain the case even when research is normalised for other contributing factors such as income, BMI, access to healthcare etc...

A **poor answer** would show little awareness of this as an issue or be unable to propose a reason why this may be the case.

A **good answer** could approach this question from one of a number of different avenues. For example, it may consider demographic factors as a result of wider social inequalities which then manifest in worse healthcare outcomes (for example, income disparities, quality of healthcare in general practice, or other factors likely to affect underlying health conditions). These are all pre-existing factors, exacerbated by covid. Alternatively, the answer could consider whether there are reasons why BAME people might be more likely to be exposed to covid. The answer could also consider if there are likely to be differences in quality of healthcare provided in response to covid. While overt or explicitly discriminatory differences are relatively rare, the candidate may propose ways in which current systems indirectly discriminate. For example, many people with moderate covid were sent home with advice to call 999 if their oxygen levels dropped so much they developed blue lips. This is something which is rarely visible in people of colour, and as such can delay them contacting medical professionals for help, or receiving treatment, leading to worse outcomes.

The **best answers** will consider a range of these factors, and may, through discussion with their interviewers move to suggestions as to how this could be counteracted, and how the medical profession should go about ensuring healthcare equality.

Q91: Will the global population continue increasing indefinitely? What factors might affect the ongoing population growth?

Growing populations, and (importantly) the areas worldwide which are experiencing population growth, is an important area to understand if working in public health and related fields. This question is asking you to go beyond simple statements which you may have picked up based on the news, and examine the way in which populations grow and the interconnected nature of the factors affecting population growth.

A **poor answer** would perhaps fail to consider any of the question in detail, giving simplified statements such as "*yes, the population would probably grow indefinitely until there was some change that meant the planet couldn't support the number of people – so there is probably a maximum that can be supported but that's based on environmental factors*". Alternatively, they may list a range of factors but in very little detail, for example "*there are loads of factors which will affect birth rate and death rate: contraception, education, access to food, poverty levels, health and disease, life expectancy factors*". Without further exploration (and a logical categorisation of such issues) it's difficult for an interviewer to know what conclusions you're expecting them to draw, or see evidence of your own critical analysis.

A **good answer** may start with a very simple statement which they can then explore logically in turn, for example "*I feel that fundamentally the population will continue increasing until the birth rate is lower than the death rate, once that balance changed to be approximately equal you'd see a stable global population*". Somewhat counterintuitively, this statement isn't actually correct (at least in the short-term), and so you should expect to be challenged by the interviewer. Even if the number of people born this year equalled the number of people who died, the world population would continue to grow for another couple of decades – why?

The **best answers** will consider this question, as well as expanding on the possible factors affecting both birth and death rate. For example, "*although the birth rate matched the death rate, the population would continue to grow because life expectancy has increased – so there will be more people making up the older age groups than there were previously – which will change the population profile as well*". Similarly, factors such as those identified above would be considered but with clear links, categories, or conclusions drawn, e.g. "*factors affecting birth rate include those which relate to ability to choose to have/not have children, such as access to contraception, as well as those which influence decisions about the number of children to have, such as infant mortality rate, poverty level, education, and gender equality issues. So I think if you were trying to influence this it would be important to start from the reasons behind choices, for example, reducing infant mortality would (perhaps counterintuitively) decrease the birth rate as well as the death rate, and might have a bigger impact than simply ensuring access to contraception*".

You can find more of a discussion on this topic (as well as the idea of 'peak child') in the work of Hans Rosling – which is worth an explore if you're interested in the intersection of statistics, big data, medicine, and public health policy.

Q92: I have just injected myself with an unknown substance. Work out what it is doing to my body by asking me simple questions.

This question is perhaps more likely at universities where you will take MMIs, rather than in a panel or Oxbridge interview. Nonetheless, many of the skills which the interviews are attempting to test are similar, and so you should prepare for some 'role play' and 'communication' type questions which may arise.

A **poor candidate** may attempt to use this question as an opportunity to display their knowledge of medical conditions, asking questions such as:

"Have you noticed any signs of arrhythmia since you injected the substance?"

While the intention behind this (and the use of technical language) may be appealing, it is important to bear in mind that these will likely get you poor answers such as a simple 'no', rather than collecting the specific data which you're seeking to collect.

A **good candidate** would ask simple questions such as *"Do you have any pain? Can you tell me where that pain is? Do you feel dizzy? Do you feel short of breath? How is your sense of touch/smell/taste/sight/hearing?"*. The value of these questions is that they quickly exclude large numbers of possibilities. They also, if arranged sensibly, contribute to your understanding without leaving room for omission. Importantly, you should avoid questions which are too vague (e.g. 'how do you feel?') as well as questions which are too specific (e.g. 'where are you in pain?') from the outset. This is because, in general, patients would answer the question as asked, so if you say 'where are you in pain?' and they aren't in pain, they often wouldn't naturally volunteer information about any sensations which aren't 'pain' such as dizziness or blurred vision.

An **excellent candidate** would begin by setting out exactly what they were asking about, a couple of simple statements such as *"You may have some soreness around the injection site, but for the time being we're going to ignore that and focus on any other sensations"* or *"I'd begin by asking you to think about how you felt before the injection, and then ask that you only mention sensations which have differed. So for example, if you had a headache this morning, don't worry about telling me about that if you still have the headache, only if its changed of got worse – is that okay?"*. Both of these will, most likely, increase the quality of the 'data' you get from the patient, and prevent you wasting time asking about 'pain' to find out it's in a 'muscle' only to find out that the muscle is in the upper arm, and they're referring to the injection site!

Q93: What is the mass of nitrogen in this room?

This question is very typical of Oxbridge interview questions in the sciences – it sets up a relatively complicated calculation, tests your ability to make 'common sense' estimations, and is incredibly straightforward to ask. The reason these questions are so popular is that the simpler the question is to ask (and therefore understand), the more level the playing field for all applicants.

A **weak applicant** might answer this by jumping straight to an estimate, 'I'm not sure, but 10/50/100kilos seems reasonable'. As with the vast majority of interview questions, they're not terribly interested in the answer but the working out.

A **stronger applicant** might begin by discussing equations or physical principles which might be related to the mass of air. Noting down the ideal gas equation, the molar mass of nitrogen, the composition of air, or the equation relating density and volume would all be suitable initial thoughts. The important point to consider here is that the weaker applicant may have thought of any (or all of these things), discarded some based on the information they have, and maybe even done a mental calculation before their statement that '10 kilos seems reasonable' – but if they have not discussed any of this with the interviewer they will receive no credit for the answer they have come to.

Once the possible areas to explore have been identified, the applicant will need to identify or estimate the relevant information they're going to need to use. This is where it helps to do some quick 'mental maths' (or 'mental biology') exercises in the weeks before your interview, make sure you know what a sensible estimate for things like mass, length, coefficient of friction, and similar would be. What is an average height and weight for a person? How much blood does a person have in their body? What are common values of pH or temperature for enzymes? (Remember – you don't need to know the answer here. A reasonable answer for the mass of a person could be anything from around 50kg to 120kgs if not higher/lower depending on the context. The key thing is that you can justify the answer you pick).

Finally, the candidate would use a sensible method to complete the calculation (e.g. volume x density).

If there was time available at the end, the applicant would then return to the question and move from calculating mass of air, to working out the mass fraction of Nitrogen – however it's important to note that (as with most questions) it's not necessary to make it all the way to a final answer to give a really strong interview performance.

Q94: Is humour a useful skill for a doctor?

Unlike some of the other question styles, in which you can be left guessing the exact skill or piece of knowledge which the interviewer is trying to examine, this particular question is more obvious. However, even though it's clear that the question is testing your understanding of the traits a good doctor should have, there are still a number of common errors or pitfalls which students fall into.

Poor candidates can often be too certain (or too 'extreme' in their answer). In this case, both *"it's absolutely an essential skill, almost the most important skill a doctor could have"* and *"I don't think so, I don't think any doctors need to have humour of one of their skills"* are lacking in nuance, and fail to examine the *reasons* that it may or may not be useful.

Good candidates would take a more nuanced and balanced approach – perhaps considering examples of times in which it may be useful, alongside times in which it wouldn't.

The **best candidates** might begin to explore what is meant by useful in this context at all. Some of the previous candidates may have focussed on whether a 'humorous' doctor is useful or inappropriate for the patient. Some other candidates may have focussed on whether humour is a useful skill for the good of the doctor, for example using dark humour in a personal setting to decompress after a situation in which they've had to break bad news, or been under significant stress. The best candidates will identify both of these possible values, and begin to explore how they're linked. If humour is a useful skill for a doctor's personal mental health, what are the knock on effects on patient care?

Importantly there is no right answer, and there are a lot of doctors who are very successful with or without this skill. However, your answer should show an understanding of both sides of an argument before coming to an overall judgement such as, *"I think it could be useful to some people on a personal level, but I think there are so many other skills which are much more essential across the board and useful for a doctor to have that although this is 'useful' its quite low importance".*

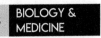

Q95: What is the most important technology available in medicine? Why? How could it be improved?

This question will differ based on your prior experience and your idea of importance. The key factor in a good answer is examining your underlying assumptions (in this case 'what makes something important?') alongside coming to an answer.

A **poor candidate** might give an example, but fail to identify why it's important or how it could be improved. For example, *"I think the most important technology in medicine is x-rays – they've just been so influential and we use them loads"*.

A **good candidate** would give an example, and make sure to include their justification – leading to an answer such as *"I think the development of genome mapping technologies is the most important technology to medicine. It has applications in improving and influencing a range of other incredibly significant therapies and public health techniques – such as the development of vaccinations, targeted individual therapies for cancer, as well as the prospect of influencing inherited conditions. I think at the moment, the biggest areas for improvement relate to speed or cost."*

The **best candidates** would show a clear examination of the criteria they're using to decide if something is important in medicine, perhaps with an initial discussion such as, *"There is such a broad range of technology available that I think it's important to first decide how I'd tell if something was important. There are a few factors, such as impact on individuals (so if something is lifesaving that's high importance), as well as impact in terms of number of people affected. Based on that I think the most important thing must be the thing that has the biggest individual impact, so is lifesaving, as well as having an impact on the largest number of people. I think that leads to technologies such as vaccines or antibiotics, based on the amount of impact they have on the world…"*

This answer could then go on to discuss the possible improvements.

Importantly, which technology you choose is unimportant provided you can (and do) clearly justify the reasons that you deemed it to be important.

Q96: If you lived in the 18th century, how would you prove that different areas of the brain have different functions?

While hypothetical, this question is testing your ability to propose sensible (and ethical) real-world experiments, as well as your understanding of how medicine as a field has developed.

A **poor candidate** may come to the conclusion that there would be no way to prove this with the technology of the time. Or may consider a range of ethical issues (in their head), but fail to include the interviewer in their thought process, and as such give a very limited answer.

A **good candidate** might propose that there is a need to have an independent variable, such as 'area of brain which is damaged' and a dependent variable, such as 'impact on behaviour, personality, or other outcome'. They may then discuss ways in which this could be tested. In the 18th century lobotomies were not uncommon, however any discussion of lobotomy for experimental purposes (particularly with the intention of damaging parts of the brain to deduce function) has quite clear issues, which should be stated!

The **best candidates** would therefore propose ways in which the same outcome could be achieved, but without needing to actively act unethically. Perhaps it would be possible to examine patients who have experienced damage to their skull or brain and create a profile of 'before' and 'after'. Importantly, top-level candidates may point out areas in which this kind of examination may introduce areas of bias. For example, if everyone who is shot in a particular part of the head dies (because that part of the brain controls unconscious systems such as breathing) then they would be excluded from data collected based on interviews with surviving brain damage patients. This is called survivorship bias, and is just one example of the kind of issues which could arise in a study such as this unless actively mitigated against.

Q97: How do archaeologists decide which fossils are 'people' and which are something earlier?

This question, initially seems disconnected from medicine (or related subjects) and therefore often poses a challenge to students who are looking for the underlying reason they're asked the question in order to figure out the *right* answer. The other challenge in this question is that you can interpret it in two different ways: either it's a question about the methods and technology which archaeologists use to categorise remains, or it's a (more relevant) question about how they decided on the categories in the first place. In other words, what makes people *people*?

Importantly, interviews aren't conducted in a vacuum, and are intended to be a discussion, so if you were to focus on a different aspect of the question that the interviewers intended that's okay – they will generally prompt you to refocus in the right direction!

A **poor answer** would fail to appreciate the meaning of the question, even with prompting to answer 'how do we decide where people start?', for example. Alternatively an answer may focus too much on things being done *'because that's how they've always been'* or, rather vaguely, *'it matches the criteria'*, without showing any critical analysis of how such criteria came to be.

A **good answer** would consider one of two key strands which could underpin a discussion of what makes a person a person, the appearance and structure of the fossils (physical characteristics), and the behaviour.

The **best answers** might begin to link both of the strands mentioned above, to discuss how behaviour affects physical characteristics (and where you might see this in someone's skeletal remains), or vice versa. They may also go on to discuss the ways in which statements such as *'humans are capable of self-actualisation'* could be explored with very limited information remaining. How can we see evidence of behaviour in fossil records (e.g. healed bones indicating a move beyond a 'survival of the fittest' mentality as a species)?

It is likely that the discussion would develop into one of a number of topical discussions more directly related to medicine. For example, 'what are our criteria for determining what a person is today?' and follow up questions about determining where human life begins, and the ethics of embryonic stem cell research for example.

Q98: How could you measure how much blood is in your body right now?

This question could, for some applicants, simply be a case of recall. If you're lucky enough to have observed a blood volume test as part of your work experience then stating your knowledge would be sufficient to answer the question. However, blood volume tests are quite rare, so for the majority of candidates this is an opportunity to develop a method all your own.

A **poor answer** may ignore the keyword 'measure' and instead propose ways in which you could calculate or estimate the amount of blood in your body. Some students focus on how much blood a person has per unit of weight on average, and as a result fail to answer the question at hand. This kind of answer, *"I'd weigh myself and then multiply weight by blood per unit weight"* also fails to show an appreciation of the uses and limitations of averages. It would simply tell you how much blood you might expect to have, or how much blood an average person who looked like you would have, but it wouldn't tell you how much *you* have personally.

A **good answer** may begin to propose ways that you could find out about blood flow, even if it isn't initially linked to an actual solution to the question. Many students begin, for example, by stating that *"you could measure the volume of blood per second in a blood test"*. Although this answer isn't fully developed, it does then give opportunities for the interviewers to prompt you (and shows you're thinking of practical methods which could be applied). Even if you're unsure how you'd find certain values, a good answer would make a note of the values which would be needed, *"In order to find the total volume of blood though, I'd need to be able to multiply that value by the total number of seconds which it takes for the blood to flow all the way around the body"*. This is valuable for two main reasons – it shows the interviewer your thinking (even if you don't reach a solution) and saying it aloud may prompt your own thought process.

The **best answers** would look broadly similar to the way in which blood volume tests are actually carried out, and suggest the use of a tracer to find the length of time taken.

The discussion may then turn to the candidates understanding of how tracers or medical imaging work, or the possible repercussions of having too much or too little blood in the body.

Q99: How do you know if someone has a mental illness? How would you tell if they didn't?

This question is asking you to consider how diagnosis works, as well as what is meant by mental 'health' and mental 'illness'. It is important when answering a question like this to attempt to examine how the criteria came to be the way they are, in order to show your analytical approach. The challenge is in balancing this analytical approach, and avoid giving the appearance that you feel you know better on every point – which is sometimes a very fine line.

In this question a **poor candidate** would give a relatively simplistic answer such as 'you'd match up their symptoms with the criteria for different mental illnesses and see what they had. You'd know if they didn't if they didn't meet the criteria'. This is a weak answer for a number of reasons, not least of which the interconnected nature of many mental illnesses mean that people will 'tick boxes' for a number of conditions. On the other hand, very few people won't 'tick one box' at any given time – but this doesn't mean that doctors should be diagnosing everyone with a mental health condition.

A **good candidate** would highlight some of these nuances and perhaps begin to bring in the idea of 'impact' as well as 'symptom'. In general, particularly when dealing with mental health, medical professional assess the extent to which a particular condition impacts the persons ability to carry out their day to day activities. This means that mental health (should) be considerably more tailored to the individual, particularly because it's more difficult to get a quantitative assessment.

The **best candidates** will begin to address the second question – how do we tell if people are mentally healthy? Importantly, they will perhaps attempt to define health v mental illness based on averages (what a 'typical person' experiences), and will raise pros and cons of their own definition. Moving on from this, they may begin to discuss the risks of over-diagnosis: if some conditions in the DSM have 'feel excessively fatigued' as a symptom, and some have 'feel like I have too much energy or I can move more quickly than normal' – where do you draw the line between illness and health?

Q100: Should we be trying to cure conditions such as autism or downs syndrome?

This question is increasingly topical and raises issues around the meaning of cure, and the difficult interactions between medical research and communities of people with autism or other neurodivergent or inherited conditions. Importantly, you should ensure that you consider both sides of the argument in justifying your conclusion, but make sure to do so in a way that doesn't seem like you're continuously changing your mind. A lot of people make the mistake of feeling that they have to present both sides of an argument entirely passively, but this can lead to confusion – so it's okay to say 'I know that the main opposing argument is… however I feel that', rather than simply listing for and against.

A **poor answer** may be simply a 'yes' or 'no' answer, or one which failed to show any appreciation of the fact this may be a 'grey area'. Answers such as *"of course we should, the point of medicine and medical research is to keep people healthy, so if we can make people healthier by curing diseases we should"* are not uncommon. However, they fail to examine what they mean by 'healthy', have an underlying assumption which is unchallenged that being on the autism spectrum is 'unhealthy', and also overlook the fact that the majority of 'cures' at the moment come in the form of pre-natal screening to allow parents to make informed choices about having children with these conditions.

A **good answer** would show an appreciation of a number of the areas highlighted above, for example: *"I think that this is probably a question which should be informed by the opinions of people with autism, or with the other conditions mentioned. Often, people with autism don't feel a cure is required, because they don't feel the condition has a negative impact on their life. However, in the case of people with autism with more significant impairments this decision would have to be made on their behalf".* They may then go onto discuss what the value of a cure is for any condition.

Q101: If a psychologically ill person commits a crime, are they a criminal?

It should be quite straightforward to identify the ethical quandary or conflict in this question, which is aiming to explore the challenge of assessing personal culpability when people have psychological health conditions. There are a few key things to remember in questions like this one. Firstly, it is important to define any assumptions on which your later reasoning lies. And secondly, there are (generally) no prizes for simply noting that this is a challenging or 'grey' area. The interviewers know this already! They're interested to see how comfortable you are drawing balanced, evidence based, and also ethically rigorous conclusion.

A **very poor candidate** may fail to recognise that this, and scenarios similar to this, are ethically challenging. While competence and confidence are important qualities for doctors, arrogance most certainly isn't. Candidates who answer this question immediately with a definite answer which lacks awareness of why this is in any way challenging, lacks empathy, or hints at internal biases would be unlikely to succeed. For examples 'yes, mental health issues shouldn't be used as an excuse to avoid fair punishment'. Although this may seem very similar to a successful answer below, the use of the word 'excuse' for example suggests some internal biases on the part of the candidate.

A **poor candidate** may simply give tangentially related examples, for example: 'This sort of question often has to be asked if defendants in criminal cases claim that they weren't sane at the time of the crime'. While this is certainly a start, and it's good that the candidate has a clear understanding of what they're being asked, this doesn't really contribute anything to answer the question, it simply reposes the question back to the interviewer.

A **good candidate** may begin by examining some of the key words in the question. For example, is a criminal simply 'one who commits a crime'? Or is the word 'criminal' inherently negative, and therefore people who commit crimes but who are deemed to have lacked responsibility for their actions at the time the crime was committed shouldn't be saddled with it. Secondly, how is psychological illness defined? Given that humans are, in general, sociable creatures and that natural selection is likely to have favoured traits which foster social cohesion, could it be argued that anyone who commits a violent crime against another person must therefore be of unsound mind? If this is the case and committing a violent crime would therefore prove, by necessity, psychological illness, how does that affect personal responsibility?

Importantly, the **best candidates** will examine the many avenues available in this question in a structured and logical way – perhaps even beginning with a statement such as 'There are clearly quite a few things to think about here – what do we mean by psychologically ill, what determines if someone is a criminal, and how they affect each other'. They would also end their answer with a *clear conclusion* based on their thought process. Importantly, you don't have to know what your answer is going to be before you start, because you can (and should) examine both sides. But your answer must follow naturally from the arguments which you stated were the most convincing throughout your discussion.

Q102: If you had to give human rights to one of either chimpanzees, dolphins or elephants, which would you choose?

As with many of these questions, you may wish to spend a brief period of time before you answer assessing *what* the question is trying to test. This question could be testing a few different areas, and you may wish to consider any of the following questions in answering: What are human rights? What characteristics of the animal in question would you use to determine their rights? Are there any ethical issues with using species characteristics to determine rights (consider if individual characteristic variation within a species was used to determine personal rights – this would widely be condemned – what's the difference?)? What benefits would there be to being given human rights? Might one of the species benefit more from being given human rights?

A **poor candidate** would give an answer which lacked a clear critical analysis of the reasoning behind their gut instinct. For example, 'I think I'd choose chimpanzees, because they're the most like humans out of the other animals'. Stating your gut instinct is not necessarily a bad thing, and candidates should be equally wary of endlessly equivocating without a clear answer. However, the issue here is that the candidate doesn't examine what they mean by 'most like humans' which significantly limits their answer. Is this based on DNA? Physical characteristics? Mental characteristics?

A **good candidate** would show an understanding of what human rights are, and the value of extending rights to certain animals or species. They would then consider each of the species in turn to decide either: which species is most deserving of human rights, or which species would benefit the most from human rights.

The **best candidates** would begin with a brief explanation of their understanding of human rights, with a focus on what human rights seek to achieve as a general principle, rather than any single right itself. For example, 'I think the main aim of human rights is to ensure people are free from suffering in a range of forms'. They would then link this to their examination of which animal would be most suitable/justified in receiving human rights. In this case, if the candidate has identified 'freedom from suffering' then they may seek to determine which animal has the greatest capacity to suffer (justification based on species characteristics), or which animal would see the greatest reduction in suffering as a result of gaining human rights (justification based on impact). They may even examine both of these justifications (which may be contradictory), prior to coming to one final answer.

Q103: Why do men often go bald, but women rarely do?

This question isn't testing your knowledge of male (or female) pattern baldness! Although it can be a bit more challenging in specific questions such as this one to see how you would go about answering if you don't *just know* the answer, it's important to bear in mind that your thought process is still important.

A **poor candidate** might be too worried about this being something they've been expected to know, and fail to propose their own answers as a result. Alternatively, they may give an answer which at its core is simply restating the question, for example, 'I think it's probably based on biological differences between different sexes'. While this isn't incorrect, and the appearance of difference between the sexes is likely biological – you can hopefully see that it isn't really contributing much to explain *why*.

A **good candidate** would make a suggestion as to what the underlying cause of this difference could be. For example, 'Baldness is probably the result of hair follicles becoming damaged, and so it seems likely that there is something which men have in their system and women don't which causes this... I think it's probably hormonal, so it could be that testosterone is damaging to hair follicles'. You should note here that the candidate quite clearly doesn't know, but is making logical (and sensible) deductions, and also brings in a small amount of their own knowledge of hormones which are found more in men than women.

An **excellent candidate** would make multiple suggestions. For example, must it be the case that testosterone is damaging hair follicles or could it be that hormones occurring in greater amounts in women (such as oestrogen) are protecting follicles in some way? Alternatively, what if it's nothing to do with 'men' as a whole (given there are a large number of men who don't go bald)? Perhaps it is worth exploring the idea that it could be inherited, and may be a mutation which occurs more frequently on the Y chromosome, and therefore has a sex-based heritability difference?

The **very best candidates** may even challenge the premise of the question (though it is worth noting that there are lots of examples of times that this would instead be a bad thing to do!). Do men actually bald more than women, or do they simply bald in different ways? Male pattern baldness generally involves follicles becoming damaged in a single large area, whereas female pattern baldness involves the distributed loss of follicles throughout the scalp (resulting in hair thinning, or patches of baldness). If, in fact, there is no difference in frequency, but rather a difference in presentation based on biological sex how does this affect any previous answers?

Q104: Why is there no cure for the common cold? How does the flu vaccine work?

Given the massive increase in public education and understanding of virus transmission and vaccination as a result of the covid-19 pandemic, it is vitally important that you show that you have an understanding of these relatively basic pillars of public health information. In contract to the majority of questions in this book, the focus in this question (which would likely be quite introductory) is not to give such an excellent answer they give you an offer, it's to avoid giving such a bad answer that you 'fail' the interview before you've really started. This is one of the few questions in which they are testing your common knowledge, rather than your thought process.

A **poor candidate** wouldn't have the biological basis to answer the question convincingly. They may focus on less relevant areas, such as 'you can't create a cure because there are too many strains of the common cold to get a cure which works for all of them', rather than the greater challenge of how you create 'cures' for virus-borne illnesses. Alternatively, they may give an overly simplistic answer to the question of vaccination such as 'vaccines mean your body is familiar with the flu, so that if you get it you can fight it off better'. This isn't incorrect – but where in 'your body' is affected by the vaccination? And what do they mean by 'familiar' or even 'fight it off'?

An **average candidate** would show a competent, if limited, understanding of both the difficulty of curing viruses, and the way in which vaccination works.

An **excellent candidate** would combine their understanding of how viruses work, how we can medically target viruses and, importantly, *human behaviour* in order to answer the question. There are a large number of strains of the family of viruses which cause the common cold, and although they don't mutate terribly regularly, it is therefore difficult to create a vaccination (or cure) which would work on such a large number of commonly circulating strains. There is also a question of motivation. Although colds are incredibly common, they're also (generally) unlikely to cause any significant symptoms, and most people recover within a few days. This means, that by the time someone could be tested to check they had a rhinovirus, they'd probably have recovered without the need for a cure. Developing separate cures for the large number of strains is also incredibly expensive, for an illness which doesn't have many consequences for the majority of the public.

Q105: What is health? What is normality?

This question is, for many candidates, surprisingly difficult to answer. It falls into the category of questions which you assume you know the answer to until you're suddenly on the spot, and it becomes much less clear-cut! Importantly, it can lead to an excellent discussion of the role of doctors – which, very simply, boils down to whether their role is to promote health or minimise ill-health.

A **poor candidate** may give a short answer which doesn't show an ability to consider any challenges or weaknesses in their statement. Importantly, making a statement such as, 'health is when someone's body is working as it would be expected to in response to standard external conditions' might not be a bad answer. However, it's important that you show your ability to challenge your own thinking, without the need for input from an interviewer. So the above definition has some potentially weak areas such as: Does this include mental health? How do we account for natural intraspecies variation in our understanding of health? How do we set our expectations (e.g. in a society with increasing levels of obesity, taking 'expected' as the average now would give a different answer to the average 50 years ago, but surely there hasn't been a biological change in that time which would account for the difference?

A **good candidate** would show an awareness of the challenge of the question and follow an iterative process in order to work towards an answer they are happy with. For example, they may begin with a statement such as 'typically, people might consider health to be the absence of disease or illness'. They would then actively challenge any weaker areas in their original statement, for example, given the number of cells in a human body it is likely that everyone has some areas working 'defectively' at all times. Does this mean no one is every healthy? If not, how would you draw a boundary between situations which would be categorised as disease or illness, and those which wouldn't? Is the difference purely biological, or is it social? We don't class baldness as an illness, but we do class blindness in that way, despite the fact both could be caused by the gradual degradation of specific types of cells – what's the difference?

Excellent candidates may build on their answer, and the discussion with the interviewers, in order to begin considering the wider implications of the difficulties in defining health on the ability of doctors to make diagnoses or prescribe treatments. They may, based on their own research, then be able to link this to real-world examples of the ways in which healthcare professionals do attempt to draw quantitative and specific boundaries between the relatively vague concepts of 'health' and 'disease'.

Q106: What is the DSM? How do you think doctors should responsibly use the DSM?

As with the vast majority of Oxbridge interview questions, testing your knowledge of the field is only a small part of the challenge. So, in questions like this, as in all questions, if you're uncertain it's much better to tell them that so they can lead the discussion and give prompts to allow you to show your understanding and problem-solving ability.

If you're unsure what the DSM is, that's okay (although perhaps worth taking a look at before your real interview!). Your interviewers would likely give you an explanation such as the one below to allow you to answer the rest of the question:

*"The DSM is the **D**iagnostic and **S**tatistical **M**anual of Mental Disorders – it was first published in 1952 to allow for standardised characterisation and classification of mental disorders by medical professionals".*

A **poor answer** might focus on one specific aspect of responsible medical practice, such as competency, and as a result fail to address the ethical issues surrounding the DSM specifically. For example, *"I think responsible use of the DSM would mean ensuring that you kept up-to-date if there were additions or adjustments, so that you know everything in there and can make sure you don't miss signs".* This is a poor answer for a number of reasons, not least of which being that the candidate shows no appreciation that if their aim in practicing medicine is to 'know everything' they're going to be sorely disappointed once they receive their first reading list. It could similarly be improved by directly linking to the professional requirements rather than just alluding to the idea of competency.

A **good answer** would get to the heart of the question being posed, and give an answer which considered both the benefits and difficulties posed by use of the DSM in practice, in order to give recommendations for how to use it *responsibly.* For example, they may begin by stating the many reasons why standardised tools for diagnosis can be beneficial, in reducing bias, aiding consistent access to care, and increasing transparency (and therefore autonomy) for patients. However, there are a number of difficulties with the approach taken in the DSM, and it is commonly criticised for pathologizing behaviours which are simply indicative of typical human behaviour when in distress. The ongoing challenges of preventing over-medicalisation would potentially also be mentioned here. The student would then bring these together to suggest checks and balances which might be in place for use of the DSM, or perhaps even the expected checks and balances for how the DSM is contributed to and rewritten based on empirical data.

Q107: Why are so few flowers and animals coloured green?

This question is testing a number of key skills in your understanding of biology: can you propose common sense reasons for adaptations, do you understand how characteristics arise, and can you link the adaptations to the purpose they serve. For many students, once they begin thinking about this question they find that they almost have too much to say. It's important to try and pre-empt your answer so that you structure your thoughts logically, and it's easy for the interviewer to draw out all of the key points you made. Think of it like planning an essay so that it lines up with the mark scheme – you want to make it really easy for them to see all of the valuable points you make.

A **poor answer** would give an answer which was limited in detail or focussed too heavily on where the green colouration of plants comes from. For example, *"flowers aren't green because they need to be colourful to attract pollinators, and animals don't photosynthesise so they don't have chlorophyll to make them green"*. None of this answer is technically incorrect, but it misses the point of *why*, particularly in the second half. Animals don't have chlorophyll – why? Given chlorophyll is so readily abundant in the plants which many animals eat, why is it not beneficial for the animals to use this in the same way?

A **good answer** would address each of the parts of the question (flowers, and animals) separately, given there are likely very different reasons. They may further break down animals into mammals, birds, lizards, amphibians given there are quite significant differences in colouring between them. In the case of animals, they may go on to discuss camouflage, and which animals are green (e.g. many lizards and amphibious animals). In this case, why is there such a discrepancy? It may be tempting to say that lizards and amphibians are commonly in green environments so their camouflage matches their surroundings, but many birds also commonly nest off the ground – why are they not green?

The **best answers** would simultaneously consider many of the points above, and bring up areas of weaknesses in their own reasoning without needing prompting from the interviews. They may also begin to consider characteristics of the predators, as well as the prey (for example, colour-blindness in many mammals), to explain the differences between mammals, birds, lizards, and amphibians.

Q108: Radiation can cause cancer, yet we commonly use radiotherapy to treat cancers. Surely this doesn't make sense?

This question doesn't rely on a great deal of knowledge of the mechanisms by which cancer replicates, or cancer treatment, although a basic understanding would be helpful.

A **poor answer** might focus too specifically on exactly why radiation is a suitable treatment for cancer in particular, and may give a very detailed answer – but just not address the underlying point.

They key point which the interviewers are trying to ask about is the fact that many therapies rely on, or actively use, the same materials which cause the disease in the first place. This is not exclusive to cancer treatment, with common side effects of many anti-depressants being depression, or arrhythmia drugs which can cause heart palpitations.

A **good answer** would extract the wider point being made, and then begin to form their answer around that. Why is it that many of the treatments we use can cause the ailment they treat? Taking cancer as an example, radiotherapy is used to disrupt the ability of the cancer cells to replicate. When radiation can cause cancer, it disrupts the genetic code in cells (often the telomeres) changing the rate and extent of replication. What are the similarities and differences here?

The **best answers** would identify that therapies have to interact with the same systems and pathways which are 'malfunctioning' in the original issue. As a result, the best treatments will often be adapted versions of the causes, given that those causes can clearly interact with the systems required (whether it's disrupting the genetic code of cells, or binding to serotonin receptors, for example). The role of the medical practitioner in these situations is to balance the harm which could be caused by the treatment, with the harm which the lack of treatment would cause. This could then lead to a more in-depth ethical discussion about decision making in medicine.

Q109: How would you find out what function a gene has in humans? What about in plants?

This question has a range of possible answers which vary from more simple and cheap options which would give a relatively imprecise answer, to incredibly expensive and complex options which involve mapping the genome of large numbers of people in full to do comparative analysis. In addition to the normal advice of not panicking if you're unfamiliar with the theory (because they're looking for whether your common sense is sensible), it's also worth ensuring you consider a range of pros and cons to the method you propose. Scientific research isn't just about getting the 'right' answer, it's also constrained by economic constraints, or limitations on ethical practice, or time constraints – you should try and consider these in any questions surrounding the development of a method for research such as this one.

A **poor answer** might make vague statements, such as 'you'd compare someone without a trait with someone with that trait and see what the difference is'. This is non-specific (what would you be comparing?), but even if it wasn't it fails to incorporate an awareness of the practicalities. For example, how many people would you need to compare to be able to ensure that the differences you identified were linked to the trait you were comparing, and not causing entirely separate differences between the people. Most importantly however, this answer approaches the question as 'how would you identify the genes responsible for certain traits?' which is easier to answer, and also subtly different. The question as asked implies that you are looking at a specific gene and trying to figure out what that does, not looking at a trait and trying to figure out the gene.

An **average answer** might correctly understand the question, but then make similarly vague attempts to answer, such as 'you could change the gene, or remove it, or replace it and see what effect that had'. With modern technology, this isn't actually as impractical an answer as it once would have been, and might be suitable in the case of research on plants, but it would pose a number of ethical issues if it was proposed for research on humans or human embryonic research. It also suffers from the same issues as the proposal above – how would you identify which difference came from the change in the gene and which was determined by other factors?

A **good answer** would show an understanding of the challenges which are posed in answering this question. Their initial suggestion might be a case of sequencing hundreds of thousands of human genomes, alongside health and characteristic data, in order to try and draw conclusions. A **very good** candidate would suggest ways this could be made more practical (it currently takes around a day to sequence an entire human genome). For example, could the code be broken down into sections based on areas where we already have some information about what it does, and then only a small region needs to be sequenced for information.

Q110: There is a test which is 99% accurate and specific (the probability of a positive test given a patient is ill is 99%, and the probability of a negative test given the patient isn't ill is also 99%). It's estimated that approximately 1% of the country have a live infection, so everyone is tested. Given that your patient gets a positive test, what are the chances they have the illness?

This question is attempting to test your attention to detail and introduce a key skill for all good scientific or medical researchers: the ability to delve into the true significance of statistics.

A **poor student** would rush through to an answer, or fail to understand the distinction between P(+ve test | illness) and P(illness | +ve test) and as a result get no further than restating the 99%. It's important to figure out how to incorporate the fact that there are actually 4 possible outcomes for any person: they have the disease and test positive, they have the disease and test negative, they don't have the disease but test positive, and they don't have the disease and test negative.

The key to this question is in spending some time understanding the probabilities and information you've been given, as well as being able to make some reasonable estimations or guesses. Drawing a diagram is a good way to summarise the information given – and while not essential, many candidates find it difficult to give a **good answer** if they don't start here (work alphabetically):

		Has the disease?		
		Yes	No	**TOTAL**
Test result?	Positive	(C) 99% of (A)	(E) 1% of (B)	(C) + (E)
	Negative	(D) 1% of (A)	(F) 99% of (B)	(D) + (F)
	TOTAL	(A) 1% population	(B) 99% population	

A **very good candidate** may then simplify this for themselves, by realising that rather than continuing to work with percentages of percentages, they could simply put a total number on the population (e.g. 100 million) to allow them to get more of a feel for what's going on in the question.

This approximation results in the following data:

		Has the disease?		
		Yes	No	**TOTAL**
Test result?	Positive	(C) 990,000	(E) 990,000	1,980,000
	Negative	(D) 10,000	(F) 98,010,000	98,020,000
	TOTAL	(A) 1,000,000	(B) 99,000,000	100,000,000

From this, the calculation of the Probability (has disease if they already have a positive test) is found by dividing box (C) by the total positive tests to give a 50% chance.

A **good candidate** would, without further prompting, make a comment on whether this seems like an answer they would have expected, and perhaps even begin to discuss the implications of this on public health responses and mass testing issues in situations such as the Covid-19 pandemic.

For further reading on this topic and apparent statistical anomaly, you may be interested in searching for 'Bayes' Theorem' online.

Q111: What is your favourite pathogen?

This question is very similar to many of the questions which you may have seen published in newspapers every year in articles asking 'How would you do in an Oxbridge interview?'. In other words, its so weird (and wonderful!) that it's actually relatively unlikely to be asked. Most questions will be academic in nature, which this one certainly isn't, or testing your familiarity with the profession and your suitability, which it also doesn't. Nonetheless, its important to have prepared for the curve-ball questions just in case, so that you can ace them and move on to the more important questions unphased.

A **poor candidate** would get too caught up on finding an exact answer, and in the case that they couldn't think of one might get stuck. It's okay to say 'I don't think I've ever really thought of this before' and then perhaps answer the related question of 'what pathogen do you think is the most interesting?'. Alternatively, the candidate might try and name something unique which they know very little about, however it's important to remember that the purpose of the interview is to display your knowledge and suitability for the course. If you can display your knowledge most effectively by talking about a relatively well known pathogen (e.g. smallpox) that would be better than trying to force a unique answer.

A **good candidate** would be able to answer, with an example, as well as an explanation of *why* that's the example they've selected. For example, they could talk about the smallpox virus and the fact it's their favourite because of its historical significance. Alternatively they may know about a particular personal favourite which is interesting because of a strange interaction it has with other pathogens (e.g. *Rhizopus microspores*) – but it really isn't essential. Other interesting pathogens include *mimivirus* which is notable for the sheer volume of genetic material found compared to the majority of viruses.

Q112: What is the difference between bacteria and viruses?

This question seems as though it's simply asking you to recall and describe content from your GCSE and A-level (or equivalent) studies. However, importantly it's an opportunity for prompts from the interviewer to test the depth of your understanding, as well as your level of interest in reading beyond the syllabus to learn more about key topics of interest.

Assuming that most candidates would give an answer which was at least scientifically correct, a **poor candidate** would limit their answer to relatively simple points. For example, *"Bacteria are alive, whereas viruses aren't so they need a host"* or *"bacteria are much bigger than viruses"*. Alternatively, they may focus on the outcomes, rather than the differences between the structures, with a statement such as *"Bacteria can be targeted by antibiotics, whereas viruses can't"*, which doesn't really answer the question.

A **good answer** would not only state information, but also delve into what their means, and why it might be the case. They would be expected to show an understanding of the grey area which surrounds the classification of viruses – if they can replicate, and when in cells can significantly impact the host organisation, why aren't they alive? They would also be able to give a detailed explanation of the structure of both bacteria and viruses – for example, do they both have a protein-based protective coating? Does this have implications for treatment?

An **excellent candidate** would, under prompting from the interviewers, begin to explore further questions, such as 'what impact do you think the classification of viruses as non-living has on research?' or 'how would you determine whether a mystery ailment was caused by a bacteria or a virus?'. Alternatively, an interviewer might lead the discussion towards the impact of bacterial pathogens v viral pathogens on human behaviour or evolution.

Q113: How does a caterpillar transform into a butterfly?

As previously mentioned, in the case of many of these questions it is really important to avoid getting too focused on the exact knowledge which you're being asked about. Fundamentally, if the interviewers wanted to test which candidates could explain metamorphosis best, it would be in their interest to give you advanced notice to research the topic. They are, therefore, not looking for knowledge but scientific *common sense* and reasonable, logical suggestions.

A **poor answer** would, most likely, fail to answer the question because the candidate felt they lacked the prerequisite knowledge, or give an answer which was incorrect as a result of their confusion, for example: *"I really don't know, I think there's probably a process which goes on where the genetic material in caterpillars retains its knowledge of what it needs to do, and that's quite different to what you see in other animals so I'm not sure how that would happen"*. The issue with this statement is that 'genetic material' 'knowing' what it needs to do is, on a simple level, what it does! Although transformation on the scale seen from caterpillars to butterflies during the life-cycle is rare, all animals undergo a vast transformation in their early development, which isn't rare at all!

A **good answer** would give a brief summary of the process as observed, and then begin to fill in details about the transformation process. For example, in order to rearrange on such a massive scale, much (but not all) of the caterpillar's body is broken down into a cellular 'soup'. How is it broken down? Which systems do you think would not be broken down because they're 'essential'? Which systems do you think reform first?

The **best answers** would draw in their knowledge of the developmental stages of other organisms in order to draw out parallels. They may also incorporate an understanding of the vulnerability posed in the transformation process, to begin to attempt to explain *why* not just *how*.

Q114: Why do some habitats support higher biodiversity than others?

In order to be able to answer this question you need to understand what is meant by biodiversity, and habitat, but beyond that this question asks 'why?' and so is looking for sensible suggestions rather than prior knowledge.

A **poor candidate** might give an answer which showed a confused, or very limited, understanding of the meaning of biodiversity, for example *"more animals can live in places where there's more food, so in habitats which lots of plants you'd get a lot of biodiversity because there are lots of animals"*. This doesn't really address the difference between number of animals of a single species, vs diversity in number of unique species present in an ecosystem. Alternatively, they may give an answer which fails to identify underlying factors and as a result is vague, or even incorrect, under further examination, such as *"it's cyclic, so the more diversity you have the more food and materials you get cycling back into the environment, the more other animals you get – so it all depends on which of the habitats had an uneven amount of animals and plants to begin with"*.

A **good candidate** would show an understanding of the ways in which a habitat influences the eco-system that develops and would show their knowledge in an organised and logical way – identifying factors such as: climate, moisture, altitude, nutrient concentration. These all contribute to the number of organisms which can be supported in a particular habitat and can increase the density of organisms significantly.

The **best candidates** would then explore why it is that particularly fertile environments (such as the rainforests or coral reefs) develop into incredibly varied and diverse ecosystems, rather than monocultures. Surely, evolution by natural selection suggests that there would be a very small number of species which were selected for over time as the *best* adapted to that environment – which would directly contradict the development of diversity. Why isn't this the case? What is the issue with this reasoning?

Q115: Why do so many animals have stripes?

Questions about adaptations, natural selection, and evolution are not uncommon at interview, because they allow interviewers to test your understanding while ensuring that they're asking about a topic which everyone should be incredibly familiar with by the time they get to the stage you're currently studying at. As a result, it can be difficult to tell how you'd differentiate yourself from other candidates in a question such as this one, which leads some candidates to overcomplicate their answers to their own detriment. There is an important balance to be struck between asking related questions to allow you to explore your own reasoning further, and ensuring you answer the question as asked.

A **poor candidate** would give an answer which mentioned the idea of camouflage, such as: *"They need to be camouflaged to avoid being vulnerable to predators, and stripes help them to blend into the background"*.

While this is a good start – there are a number of areas which may need considering to make this into a **good answer**:

- If camouflage is needed to protect against predators, why do tigers have stripes? (A commonly forgotten aspect of adaptation in interview answers is the need for predators to adapt to successfully catch their prey just as much as prey adapts to avoid predators).
- Why would stripes help them blend in? Zebra are black and white in an environment which is neither black nor white – is 'blending' really the aim here?
- Why are the stripes almost always vertically oriented rather than horizontal?
- What about stripes on animals which aren't there to make animals blend in, but rather to make them stand out – such as on wasps, bees, or hornets?

The **best answers** will answer many, if not all, of these questions in a logical order. They will make suggestions for how to reconcile the fact that stripes in certain situations are used to make animals stand out, and in others are apparently protective. For example, in the case of zebras, the stripes are quite clearly not going to help the animals blend into the background if they're stood on their own. But what if they're part of a herd of other zebra, then will they blend in? One of the key points to be made in this answer is the fact that hard edges aren't generally found in nature, and so stripes make it very challenging to see the edge of any one individual, which has various benefits.

Q116: Here's a cactus. Tell me about it.

"Tell me about it" questions can, initially, seem particularly challenging. It's not a typical interview problem of not being able to say anything, for most candidates, the problem is knowing where to start. Although it can be tempting to try and second guess the interviewers and begin answering questions they haven't asked – it's important to bear in mind that they will prompt the discussion in the direction they want it to go in, and so a 'brain-dump' of all the information you can think of is, unusually, very appropriate as a method of starting your answer here.

A **poor answer** is normally a result of the candidate lacking confidence in their ability to say anything sufficiently complicated, and as a result feeling unable to say anything. Alternatively, they may say a few reasonable comments (*'it's green', 'it's got spines rather than leaves'*) but in a particularly disorganised way which makes it difficult for the interviewer to lead the discussion in any one particular direction.

A **good answer** would perhaps follow a structure of going from high level to more specific comments, or be divided up to first look at describing the features, followed by the reasoning. An important point to make here is that it's essential you *only* describe something you can see, as far as possible. A key skill in medicine is avoiding jumping to conclusions and favouring specificity in language. For example, 'they were having a heart attack when they arrived' is a lot less useful a statement than 'they presented with a sharp pain in their left arm, and chest, and developed ventricular fibrillation within two minutes of arrival'. The same is true in this question (to a smaller extent).

The **best answers** will summarise a great deal of information into a clear and easy to understand answer, in which comparisons with similar (and different) presentations in other plants are drawn, as well as reasoning given for the adaptations which doesn't excessively distract from the question at hand.

Follow up questions about adaptations, or even questions such as 'how do you know this isn't an animal?' or 'if I begin pulling the spines off, would the cactus feel pain? How can you be sure?' may be expected here.

Q117: If you could save either the rainforests or the coral reefs, which would you choose?

This question may seem a little out of place in a medicine interview, being only tangentially related to your understanding of biology, and more obviously suitable for environmental scientists, biologists, or geographers. However, it has many parallels with real-life ethical dilemmas which the medical community have to deal with on a regular basis. It's important to bear in mind, therefore, that there is no right answer, and the interviewers aren't terribly interested in your knowledge of rainforests or coral reefs either. The most important word in the question here is *choose*. You need to show a clear methodology for your choice, and a justification of the reasons that choice was made – the result of the choice is largely irrelevant.

A **poor candidate** may give an answer such as *"I'd definitely save the rainforests because they've got loads of my favourite animals in, like orangutans"*, or alternatively, *"I don't even know how I'd begin to choose here, they both contribute so much to the environment around the world, I suppose probably the coral reefs are more significant just"*. Neither of these show a particularly strong reasoning, if any, and so regardless of whether the second candidate considered a wide range of factors – the interviewer would see them both as similarly lacking in substance.

A **good candidate** might still begin by commenting on how hard it would be to make a decision, but would then lay out a range of decision factors which they might use to make the decision. It may be appropriate to consider the effect of their decision on any of the following (which broadly fall under social, economic, and environmental categories), though there are many more:

- Air quality
- Water quality
- Global warming
- Global food supply
- Economic issues (e.g. national/international tourism)
- Biodiversity
- Scientific research opportunities (e.g. new medicines developed)

Importantly, candidates should try to layout the criteria which they're going to use to examine which of the habitats is more worth saving *before* they begin their answer, to show a clear reasoning.

The **best candidates** will, when they're developing their criteria, examine the biases or core principles (e.g. reducing suffering, ensuring environmental sustainability, minimising effect on people) which are underlying their issues. For example, some answers might suggest that as long as they knew which habitat supported the greatest number of animals, then they would pick that one. However, better answers would go further to examine whether all animals should be given equal weighting. The rainforests are home to a number of higher primates. If the aim of this particular candidate was to reduce animal suffering – would they see a greater reduction by saving a smaller number of primates, than a larger number of fish?

Q118: Is it easier for organisms to live in the sea or on land?

As with many of the comparison questions previously discussed in this book, it's important that candidates start this question with an understanding of the purpose of the question, so that they can set the priorities for their answer. The interviewers are, largely, not intending to test your knowledge of the sea or the land, and so giving excessive details about either would limit the success of an answer. Instead, the key word to draw out from this question is *easier*. As a result, you must spend time showing which factors you're examining to determine what is meant by ease, rather than delving into your understanding of marine ecosystems, for example.

A **poor candidate** would either jump directly to an answer without considering a range of factors, such as *"It's easier for animals to live in the sea because the water supports them, which is why whales can get so big and live so long"*, or they may fail to commit to a decision either way, but without demonstrating the way they might try to make such a decision.

A **good candidate** would identify a few metrics which could be used to determine what 'easier' meant, these could be qualitative (e.g. 'quality of life'-analogous measures) or quantitative (e.g. 'life-expectancy'-analogous measures), and may include any of the below:

- Availability of food
- Availability of shelter
- Number of young surviving to maturity
- Number of species (if there are more does that mean it's easier?)
- Number of organisms
- Human impact

The **best candidates** would critically evaluate the value of any measures they proposed in determining which was easier. Many of the factors identified above are incredibly species-dependent, so it's difficult to use them for a fair comparison. Alternatively they may show evidence of developing on the factors they're thinking about as they talk through their answer with the interview – for example, is 'number of young surviving to maturity' actually what they'd like to compare, or would 'percentage of young' be more indicative?

Q119: Why do only some lions have manes?

Another adaptation question, but this one explores sexual dimorphism specifically. Although you don't need to know any specifics of sexual dimorphism to be able to answer this question, any knowledge you do have will give you a head start here.

A **poor candidate** might fail to identify which group of lions have manes, and which don't. Alternatively they may identify that there is a division along sex lines but then give an erroneous reasoning, for example 'male lions have manes so that when they're hunting it protects their neck from attack'.

An **average candidate** might draw some reasonable conclusions with an answer such as:

"Male lions have manes and females don't, so it seems like it could be used to show off to attract a mate, where the female lions will select the males with the nicest manes".

This is definitely the right line of thought to be considering, however without further exploration it is insufficiently detailed.

A **good candidate** would build on the answer above and begin to delve into the question of *why*. Why would the lions mane be an indicator that female lions used when choosing a mate? This is important, because the females will be attempting to choose a mate which is most likely to have strong offspring – why would their mane be able to show any information about that?

To answer these questions, the candidate may discuss ways that the mane could be an indicator of health (for example based on colouring, size, etc...). The **best candidates** might consider that given the conditions lions live in, a large mane may directly make survival harder (by causing lions to overheat), and therefore only the strongest lions would be able to grow the biggest manes, which would be reason for selection.

A follow up question from the interviewers may consider the recorded cases when female-only prides of lions have begun to develop manes. What might be the reasoning behind this?

Q120: How many millilitres of beer (5% alcohol by volume) would an average person have to drink to be above the legal limit of 50mg alcohol / 100 ml of blood?

Calculation questions, particularly those which put the calculation in context, are not uncommon in Oxbridge interviews. You may not be given complete information to carry out the calculation, and so you must ensure that you have the confidence to make reasonable estimations or educated guesses to fill in numbers where they are unknown.

A **poor answer** might begin with some calculations (e.g. if it's a 300ml bottle of beer, that would be 15ml alcohol), but then fail to link these to the answer being sought, or the information in the question.

With many calculation questions it can be valuable to start at the answer and work backwards, it can also be valuable to plan a method 'I would calculate this, once I had that, I would be able to find this' prior to putting numbers in so that you don't get lost calculating numbers and eventually lose sight of what you know and what you have yet to find.

A **good answer** might therefore begin at the end, and consist of something like:

"If we know how much alcohol an average person is allowed per 100ml of blood, I'd first need to use how much blood they have to get a number for the total amount of alcohol they could have in their blood."

Assuming that the average person has 5L of blood, the total alcohol in their blood at the legal limit is $\frac{50\text{mg}}{100\text{ml}} \times \frac{5\text{L}}{100\text{mL}} = 2{,}500\text{mg} = 2.5\text{g}$

"Once we know the amount of alcohol in their blood, we could try to work out the amount of alcohol they ingested by estimating how much alcohol is absorbed"

Here, the candidate might make an estimate for the amount of alcohol they'd expect to be absorbed, this is likely to be based on nothing more than intuition. Candidates might say anything from 1%-100% (though most settle around 10-20%). This would lead to an amount of alcohol ingested of, for example, $\frac{2.5g}{20\%} = 12.5g$

"Then, when we know how much alcohol has been ingested, we can probably assume it has a similar density to water – so we'd get 1g = 1ml, meaning we can work out how much of the beer they'd have drunk.

Here, the 12.5g calculated previously, is converted to 12.5ml pure alcohol, which then becomes $\frac{12.5ml}{5\%} = 250ml$ total amount ingested.

The **best candidates** would follow a similar procedure to the one above, but would be able to identify areas where their assumptions were leading to over- or under-estimates, as well as making a comment on their final answer, or ways in which the calculation could be made more accurate, for example:

• How accurate is the 20% absorbed figure? What would be the effect if 100% of alcohol is absorbed, or only 1%?

• How reasonable does the final answer seem?

• How could we take into account the fact that alcohol isn't instantaneously absorbed? What would the rate of absorption mean for the calculation?

• While the alcohol is being absorbed, alcohol which is already in the blood is being metabolised into other substances? Could this rate be added?

• What would be the impact of including absorption rate, and the rate at which the alcohol is broken down into the final calculation?

Q121: Why can't you breathe underwater through a 1-metre straw?

This question is a good chance to demonstrate test an applicant's ability to think laterally and "out loud". Clearly it is not a "typical" medical interview question and you would not be expected to have pre-rehearsed an answer for this. This is by design, as the interview will often move away from purely factual recall questions to start stretching an applicant's thinking and check how well you understand fundamental concepts. Therefore, for these types of questions, you will need to be creative and use the scientific knowledge acquired from GCSEs and A-levels and apply it in an unfamiliar scenario.

A **good applicant** may start off with a jovial comment such as "Hmm, I have seen that happen a lot in movies but I guess there would be a couple of factors that would make this impossible". In the likely case that you have not thought about this scenario before, you would then be best suited to start suggesting a *few* ideas. It is better to start broad and pitch a couple of ideas if you are unsure, than to only suggest one and rigidly stick to that. An applicant could also talk through the situation step-by-step to buy some time and come up with ideas instead of sitting in silence, for example "Ok so I know that water is denser than air and I also know that the deeper you go, the more pressure there is on our bodies". This helps show the logical progression of thoughts, and can allow the interviewer to guide and help the applicant work through the situation, much like how a supervision runs. This could then lead on to an answer that talks about how to breathe through a straw you would need to suck air out of the straw but at the higher pressures it would be harder to use intercostal muscles push your rib cage up and out to draw the air in. You could even mention factors such as the water pressure maybe collapsing the straw depending on the material it is made of, in order to be comprehensive. You could even mention the length of the straw (1m) and how a tidal volume (500ml) means that you might end up rebreathing a fraction of the air you exhaled and the possible consequences of that. A good candidate will talk through various ideas, even if they later might decide some are not relevant, instead of sitting in silence until they come up with the "right" answer.

A **poor applicant** may respond that they have not covered this in their academic curriculum so far so they do not know. They might also miss the wording of the question and engage with whether it is possible or not (despite being given the information that it is not). This question is clearly not testing rote factual recall, and so not encountering this specific scenario should not mean you cannot at least suggest some ideas or put forward initial thoughts based on things you have learnt about breathing.

Q122: What is the difference between meiosis and mitosis?

This question involves slightly more factual recall than others, and unlike many questions there is clearly a right answer. However, it is not only what you say, but *how* you say and how you present it; it is important to structure your answer and not just list everything you know about meiosis for a while and then everything you know about mitosis. The question is asking for the *difference* so you would need to use comparative language in your answer

A **good applicant** might start off by briefly stating the obvious - that they are both types of cell division. They would then take a couple of points and start comparing between the two, for example, "in terms of the cell division itself, meiosis has two stages whereas mitosis has one. Regarding the outcome, mitosis produces diploid cells (46 chromosomes) whereas meiosis produces haploid cells (23 chromosomes). Mitosis produces two identical daughter cells whereas meiosis produces four genetically different daughter cells". They could elaborate on why this is make sense due to the different "roles" or requirements of cell division – meiosis needing to create variety for gametes whereas mitosis being used in repair and growth so an exact copy is more ideal. Note how there is a constant back-and-forth comparison between the processes to help illustrate what the differences are, and the opportunity to begin to touch on why this difference is needed.

A **poor applicant** might think of this as a chance to "brain dump" all the things they know about this topic in a textbook-style manner by talking about mitosis and listing all the stages in great detail (prophase, prometaphase, metaphase, anaphase, and telophase). They would then probably do the same for meiosis. However, although that shows good recall, the question has not been specifically answered. It is understandable to want to fall back on a solid ground of knowledge when answering questions under pressure but applicants should make sure that they always take a few seconds to listen and understand how the question is phrased and tailor their answer instead of only hearing keywords like "meiosis" and "mitosis" and spending minutes just purely regurgitating facts about the individual processes.

Q123: Genes - why are we not more like bananas?

A common trivia fact is that we share (around) 50% of the same DNA as bananas – you are not expected to know the exact figure and could ask the interviewer if you were unsure what the ballpark percentage is. The idea behind this question is not to recall the exact amount of DNA we share with bananas, but to explain *why* two things can share so much DNA yet be very dissimilar. This topic is covered in Biology specifications, and includes the concepts of non-coding DNA, which tests whether you have a secure appreciation for the difference between genes and DNA.

A **good applicant** would make a quick point or two about how genes are a hereditary unit made up of DNA. However, in this question, the main points to address are the difference between DNA and protein products, and the proportion of DNA that actually codes for these protein products. This can lead to discussion about how DNA itself is the sequence of bases, but only a small fraction encodes for proteins. Therefore, two organisms can share a lot of the same DNA but be very different due to differences in their protein-coding exons. Drawing a quick diagram for the stages between DNA to protein synthesis can help show an applicant's understanding of the process and how some (and in fact the vast majority of) DNA is not involved in this. This can lead onto a discussion of possible functions of the DNA that does not encode proteins, and the applicant should be comfortable suggesting regulatory roles or codes for RNA that can control cellular reactions.

A **poor applicant** might have a weaker understanding of the concept of genes and think they are synonymous with DNA, something which will be apparent to the interviewer upon asking this question. This will undoubtedly make it a challenge to explain why we share much DNA with a banana, but the proteins coded for are clearly different. It is important that applicants understand what they learn on a fundamental level, and that they do not only learn concepts superficially for exams.

Q124: Why do we need lungs?

This tests a fairly common topic taught at GCSE and A-level Biology so all applicants ought to be able to attempt some sort of answer to this question. The purpose of asking this question is to probe and check whether you understand the topics you have learnt, or if you have simply learned a textbook definition off-by-heart. In preparation for Oxbridge interviews, it is highly advisable that you go through and check your understanding of the key topics you have been taught as these are often used as the prompt for further questioning. Asking the "why" questions behind these concepts is a good way to assess this and often feature in interviews.

A **good applicant** will start off by explaining why we need lungs – to help with gas exchange. The term "gas exchange" is commonly associated with the lungs in exams and textbooks but it is useful to clarify what this means; helping transfer oxygen from the air into red blood cells, but also helping the body get rid of carbon dioxide. However, simply stating what the lungs do, does not fully answer the question as the applicant needs to address what is it in particular about the lungs that makes it such an important site for gas exchange. In other words, *why* we need lungs to do this. This would lead on to discussions about how the lungs use a large surface area and very thin walls to allow diffusion to take place at a rate that will meet the needs of the body. It is this adaptation that fully explains why we *need* lungs. As is often the case, a diagram drawn while talking can often help explain points and demonstrate a thorough understanding of the structures involved; if there is a pen and paper offered, do not be afraid to make use of them. Going further, an interesting way to approach this answer would be to talk about conditions where lung function is compromised and how this affects the body negatively, thus showing the need for lungs (including asthma and COPD).

A **poor applicant** might simply say "to breathe" or something similar but not actually explain what is it about lungs specifically that enables this. This shows a poorer understanding of the subjects they have encountered, and does not demonstrate as much academic interest as an applicant who takes initiative and personally makes sure they understand the topics they are learning beyond the scope of hitting marks on a mark scheme.

Q125: Why are people obese?

Obesity is an ever-growing strain on healthcare and as an aspiring medic you would be expected to have some familiarity with its effects. This question asks what *causes* obesity, which is not a particularly challenging or obscure topic to tackle in terms of content, but requires a structured answer to cover a wide range of causes. Importantly, an interviewer would be looking to make sure that the applicant appreciates that there are often multiple factors at play and this is not often attributed to one cause.

A **good applicant** would begin by briefly addressing what obesity is and how to define it (commonly stated as a BMI that is greater than 30). This does not take into account a bodybuilder's physique, and it is fair for you to say you will be only considering obesity as cases when a person has this BMI due to excess fat. A good way to structure the answer would be to look at the "intake" and "expenditure" causes as when energy intake exceeds expenditure, there will be weight gain. From the intake angle relevant factors include; bigger portions, eating "unhealthy" (fried, high calorie) fast food regularly and poorer food choices. It is also important to mention that this is not always due to a person being "lazy", but there can be socioeconomic or mental health issues at work. For example, it is often cheaper to eat unhealthy fast food than to buy healthy meals when out and about. As a potential future medic, it is important not to seem like you are implying that obesity is always a choice and the person is solely to blame. On the expenditure side of things factors include; a sedentary lifestyle, lack of exercise, genetics and states of disease (for example, thyroid function disorders). Again, this changes the element of culpability and highlights factors beyond a person's control in some cases. It would be interesting to mention the recent increasing trends in some of these factors and why this means more people are becoming obese and at a younger age, which would help support your points as being causative in nature. Overall a good applicant will realise the multifactorial nature of obesity, and will be able to express this is in a logical and structured manner.

A **poor applicant** might not realise all the factors that come into play and may simply say "eating too much and not exercising enough". This neglects the element of individuality from person to person, for example, thyroid disorders may mean two people who do the exact same activities and eat the same foods can have different weights. From a prospective medical student point of view, it is important to tackle this issue of culpability and a poor applicant may place most of the "blame" on the individual and not realise the wider socioeconomic causes of why some people are obese and the health crisis we face.

Q126: How does a bird fly?

This question does not address a topic covered in most Science specifications and therefore tests the applicant's ability to think laterally with information they do know in an unfamiliar context. The need to do this is very typical of an Oxbridge interview and you should be comfortable with trying to extend your thinking into areas you may not have "rehearsed" for. Everyone has a basic understanding that birds flap their wings to lift off and this question asks you to engage with this aspect from the perspective of basic BMAT-level Physics to come to an explanation of how this works.

A **good applicant** will take the situation step-by-step to explain how birds can fly. During take-off, birds unfold their winds and create a down stroke which compresses the air beneath their wings. If an interviewer gives you this first step as a clue, you should realise that this compression results in increased air pressure and helps thrust the bird upwards. By flapping their wings (hence the need for strong breast muscles) they achieve the forward thrust needed to direct their flight, whilst air rushing against the wings helps maintain the vertical lift. Finally, gliding is achieved due to a streamlined body and wings, which you should realise will result in less air resistance. You could draw on the similarity between how a plane flies to help explain your answer, mentioning that the engine is what is used to thrust planes into the air and explain the parallel mechanism seen in birds. An additional angle you could mention in your answer are further adaptations that make it possible for such mechanisms to work. Some examples include hollow bones (which reduce their weight) and light feathers (to catch the air).

A **poor applicant** might respond with an overly simplistic answer, for example "with their wings" but be unwilling to pursue this any further for fear of being wrong. This fails to appreciate the fact that the question is not testing conventional factual recall, but asks the candidate to think creatively using basic concepts they do know and further clues from the interviewer. In these types of interview questions, the worst thing to do is to be scared of "getting it wrong" and to not engage at all as this suggests the supervision style of learning is not one you will thrive in.

Q127: What is the relationship between flow through a vessel and its diameter?

This question tests a basic physiological concept that the applicant has likely encountered before, or can otherwise logically work out. This phenomenon of flow and diameter has important relevance in the field of Medicine when thinking about blood flow through various vessels in the body and how this can be altered in disease. It is appropriate for interviewers to evaluate whether applicants can understand and grasp such an important concept, and to see their thought processes in how they try to logically work out the relationship between the two parameters.

A **good applicant** will start out with facts that they do know and then start working out additional conclusions from there on. It is reasonable to assume that as the diameter increases, so does the cross-sectional area and thus the flow increases - and this is a good place to start. However, candidates with a good grasp of basic Physics and Biology will quickly realise that this is not necessarily a linear relationship, a clue which may be given or hinted at by the interviewer. It is important to pick up on cues when the interviewer tries to help you as they are often engaging in a form of teaching where you strive to arrive at an answer of your own with some guidance. When thinking about what "hinders" blood flow (resistance), it can be deduced that this is largely from the vessel wall. However, the bigger the diameter, the lower the proportion this vessel wall makes up in comparison to the internal diameter. Thus, it can reasonably be deduced that the flow is exponentially related to the diameter. In fact, this makes up part of the Poiseuille equation, which talks about resistance to flow. If asked about this in terms of making a link to blood flow in the body, you could talk about vessels of different sizes for example capillaries versus large arteries, but then also allude to the fact that there are other factors that will determine flow.

A **poor applicant** will perhaps realise that flow will increase as the diameter increases, but will be unable to extend any deductions beyond there. Without recognising the difference between linear and exponential relationships, it would be hard for an applicant to engage with the question further and they may be unable to think creatively beyond this simplistic answer. The term "relationship" is specifically vague and it is better to think through your approach out loud even if you consider that stating this may not be linear is an obvious point not worth mentioning, as an interviewer could then hear you touch on the relevant next step to an answer and help guide you.

Q128: What is a pulse?

"Pulse" is a commonly used term in Biology and most, if not all, applicants will be familiar with the word on some level. The interviewer will use this as a basis to ask some probing questions to see if you have a solid understanding of the way the heart works, in order for you to be able to make the necessary links between how the pulse is actually generated from the heart beating.

A **good applicant** will not neglect elementary points and will start with an explanation that the pulse is equivalent to the heart rate, in other words it is the frequency at which the heart beats. However, in the context of a medical interview, it is reasonable to assume that this needs to be explained further from a physiological stance. The applicant could start by discussing where you can often feel a pulse as this is common knowledge; in the wrist or in the neck. From there, they can logically deduce that what they are actually feeling is the rhythmic dilatation of an artery. This would make the applicant think about what generates this dilation, and how this links in with the heart beating. From there it is possible to propose that when the heart contracts in systole, pressure waves are generated which moves the blood forwards and pushes arterial walls (which you will have been taught are pliable) outwards. This movement, in concert with the heart contracting (beating), are what we observe in the commonly encountered peripheral pulse. This may prompt the applicant to make further comments about why pulses will not be felt in veins, thus showing a full understanding of what the pulse is.

A **poor applicant** will probably realise that the pulse is equivalent to the heart rate but will be unable to comment further about how it is generated. Simply saying it is the heart rate is not enough as this does not explain why we have a pulse or explain what we are actually feeling when we check for the pulse as it is clearly felt in positions other than over the heart. Pushing beyond basic definitions is important, even if some answers are wrong initially, and you should start to get comfortable with suggesting ideas you are not fully sure about, but could support with reasonable and logical deductions from basic facts that you do know.

Q129: How does blood get back from your feet to your heart?

This question tests a basic understanding of the circulatory system, which is something covered both in GCSE and A-level Biology. It is not asking for the fine details about the route via names of individual veins of the leg but assesses whether you know the broad structure of a vein and how this affects the mechanics of them working under the influence of gravity. Most applicants will realise that this scenario involves venous return to the heart, but the question is asking you to consider how this travels against gravity upwards to the heart (instead of asking about an organ that is situated above the heart). Therefore, to answer the question well, you need to reference both the structure of the veins (including the valves) and the muscle contractions from skeletal muscles in the legs. As seen below, an impressive applicant will be able to link malfunction of this system to the consequence of blood pooling in the veins.

A **good applicant** will quickly realise this question is talking about veins that have come from capillary beds which need to return to the heart due to the closed nature of the circulatory system in humans. Thus, they will not be carrying blood that is pumped at high pressures generated by the aorta (as this would have damaged the capillaries) and therefore the body needs to employ a mechanism to get the blood to travel up against gravity. Simply stating the seemingly obvious challenge (travelling against gravity) shows a good understanding of the circulatory system and should not be skipped. The explanation will follow along the lines of veins having valves to ensure the flow of blood occurs in one direction (back to the heart). When we walk or get up, the skeletal muscles in our legs squeeze the veins and force the blood to move (from an area of higher pressure down a gradient) and due to the valves the only direction possible is to the heart. It would be impressive to independently back up such an explanation with an example of where this can "go wrong" although this may be a follow up question the interviewer can ask. For example, if the valves in the veins malfunction, blood can fall back downwards after every contraction and can begin to pool and cause veins to swell with blood (look up "varicose veins" if you are interested in this).

A **poor applicant** may have a flawed understanding of the circulatory system and discuss arterial flow of blood, which is not relevant to this question. Additionally, the applicant may incorrectly state that the heart pumps powerfully enough to combat gravity. Again, this shows a poor basic grasp of the circulatory system as if blood has passed through a capillary bed, the pressure from the heart's contraction will not be maintained to those necessary levels without damaging the finer structure of the capillary.

Q130: Why is blood red when you bleed even though your veins look blue?

This question is testing a commonly encountered topic in Physics; wavelengths of light. Even if you are unaware of the exact answer, this question allows an assessment of how flexible you can be with your thinking and adapt to moving away from commonly given answers relating to deoxygenated blood, which the interviewer may prompt you to discard as an avenue to go down. Stronger applicants will be able to think about other factors involved in light perception, namely the penetration of different wavelengths, whereas weaker applicants will be less able to suggest other options. It is important to pick up from cues from the interviewer and be able to be creative in the approach to answering questions if you are told you are thinking along the wrong lines.

A **good applicant** will astutely realise that if blood in veins bleeds red (as stated in the question), the colour change is unlikely to be due to the composition of the blood, as this will not change when you bleed. When suggesting answers, the applicant may mention the idea of our perception of the blood in the veins being different, to which the interviewer may encourage pursuit of reasoning. With knowledge acquired from GCSE Physics, a good applicant will be able to explain that red and blue light have different wavelengths. With encouragement from here, it is possible to deduce that these wavelengths are absorbed and reflected with different degrees of success. From the GCSE knowledge that the colour we see is what is reflected, skin and subcutaneous fat absorb more red light than blue so only the blue light is able to penetrate to our veins and be reflected back out or skin to be perceived.

A **poor applicant** might rigidly stick to the answer that veins look blue because they often carry deoxygenated blood. This is a common misconception and an interviewer would probably be prepared to hear this but then give a prompt to approach along a different line of thought, especially as the question tells us that blood is red even when you bleed through veins. Therefore, the applicant should be able to move away from the theory about deoxygenated blood. Those who fail to realise this, even with some cues, and continue to suggest this answer will fail to gain many marks or be able to make much headway with this question.

Q131: How can you stand upright and balanced even with your eyes closed?

This question is testing the foundation behind a clinically used neurological examination called Romberg's test. This is based on the fact that a person requires at least two of the following three senses to maintain balance whilst upright: vision, vestibular function and proprioception. Clearly, applicants are not expected to know this or some of the specialist terminology however through understanding how negative feedback loops work (a fundamental concept in homeostasis) it should be clear from the question that vision is an important part of maintaining balance. Furthermore, by the wording of the question, it is fair to expect you to be able to deduce that vision must not be the only sense required, and you should think rationally to suggest other mechanisms for maintaining balance. By asking this question the interviewer can assess whether you can understand basic concepts such as neuronal integration of inputs, and suggest other sources for the brain to maintain balance apart from vision.

A **good applicant** would perhaps not know the exact names or natures of the other sensory inputs, but would be willing to make guesses and try to work them out. Clearly having two feet on the ground provides some sort of sensory input that can lead to the deduction of proprioception which allows the recognition of one's position in space. Hearing is often mentioned in terms of balance in Biology specifications, and this would help lead an applicant to suggest that the auditory system plays a role in maintaining balance. By going through the other senses (such as taste and smell) the applicant can systematically decide which inputs will be relevant or not and arrive at some sort of informed answer. This shows a good understanding of how multiple inputs can be integrated in the nervous system and that this has an advantage to maintaining a function when one input is lost.

A **poor applicant** would not understand that the question relates to the nervous system and may be unwilling to suggest an answer via a systematic evaluation of the senses they have come across in their learning so far. Often these questions take key concepts learned at GCSE and A-level, and apply them to situations that applicants may not have considered before. Therefore, even if the answer is not immediately obvious, it is important to think about what principles the scenario is addressing and purely stating that you "have not encountered this before so do not know" would not be satisfactory.

Q132: How would you break the news to a farmer that his cow has died?

This question is testing your communication and empathy skills in a "breaking bad news" format. Although it is unlikely that most applicants have been in this situation themselves, you should adapt the principles of how to break bad news to this context. The interviewer is not expecting you to go into the nuances of how the cow has died, how this will affect the farmer's farm etc., but will be looking out for key skills such as sensitivity and empathy, which are obviously important for a doctor to possess.

A **good applicant** will recognise that the farmer may be upset emotionally by this news, and will demonstrate sensitive communication and empathy. A good starting point would be to initially set the scene – sit the farmer down in a quiet place, and maybe see how he thinks the cow is doing (presuming the cow has been sick for a while). A "warning shot" for bad news would be appropriate, perhaps by saying "unfortunately I have some bad news for you" to allow the farmer to prepare himself. The next step would be breaking the news and allowing a pause for the farmer to comprehend the information and react. Finally, empathising with the farmer would be important and offering support in any way that is appropriate, for example, helping with breaking the news to others. In this way, the applicant has shown that they know the key steps for how to communicate in this type of scenario, which is often tested at medical interviews.

A **poor applicant** would not realise that this is a case of "bad news" and might be too brash and come across as apathetic. It is important for doctors to demonstrate empathy and communicate sensitively with patients as different people react differently to news; what might be completely fine for one person to receive, can also be very challenging to another. Therefore, even though the applicant may not find this scenario personally upsetting, they ought to consider that the farmer may feel differently. It is also important to explicitly detail *how* to communicate, for example some mention of pausing or non-verbal communication, even if it appears obvious to the applicant.

Q133: Explain the respiratory system using this snorkel.

Clearly this answer cannot be rehearsed and the point of this task is to firstly test how well the applicant understands the respiratory system, and to secondly test how well they can create analogies of key concepts with a snorkel. The latter ensures that applicants are not simply regurgitating textbook-style answers, but actually understand the basic processes and concepts at work to the extent that they can see where parallels arise. It is important not to be phased by these more "weird" tasks, and if you get stuck to talk through how a snorkel works whilst linking back to the key concepts of the respiratory system and drawing as many creative parallels as possible.

A **good applicant** may acknowledge the odd nature of the challenge, but will not be too phased by its unpredictability and realise this question has been made unpredictable by design. They will be comfortable with picking up the snorkel and pointing to different parts and not shy away from this aspect of the task. For example, the tubes could be used to represent airways; if there is a ribbed section this could be used to explain the cartilaginous rings that prevent airway collapse at low pressures. The air inside the tube could be used to explain the concept of dead space. In this way, various creative methods can be used to explain key concepts in the respiratory system, even when the parallels are not always direct translations, have flaws and need some degree of adaptation or imagination. As long as they make sense scientifically, a good applicant will not worry that a certain parallel seems trivial and will be confident enough to mention it.

A **poor applicant** may be startled by the nature of this brief and resort to a comfort zone of purely explaining what the respiratory system via the recall of basic definitions they have learnt. This is clearly not what is asked of the applicant, and shows an inability to adapt key concepts and come up with analogies. A poor applicant may also simply describe how breathing through a snorkel works which, again, is not what is being asked of them. Even if the task seems like a curveball, it is important to realise that it is likely designed to be this way and avoiding the challenge in place of talking about something which you are more comfortable with will not be a good solution.

Q134: What is the point of cellular compartmentalisation?

Cellular compartmentalisation by membranes is a key topic covered in Biology A-levels. This question assesses whether you have a good understanding of the structure of cells and learn proactively; not just factually learning about what cellular compartmentalisation is, but *why* it is necessary. As is often the case, when going through your learning, asking these "why" questions is very important to consider. Even if an applicant has not thought about this before, it is possible to go through key functions and processes in the cell and work out why these cannot all take place in the same compartment. If there is a pen and paper available, this would be a great chance to draw a diagram to help explain what area of compartmentalisation you are talking about. Crucially, this question asks for what the point is/why it is necessary – if an applicant can only talk about what compartmentalisation is, but not why it might be necessary, the question highlights a practice of rote learning without a deeper level of understanding of cellular structures and processes.

A **good applicant** would briefly mention that cellular compartmentalisation is often achieved via the use of membranes around different organelles with controlled transport across the barriers. However, they would spend the bulk of their time talking about *why* they are needed (as the question asks) as opposed to *how* they are made. In fact, by looking at the different compartments in the cell (for example, mitochondria, Golgi, nucleus) it is clear that compartmentalisation allows many subcellular processes to occur at once by allowing required components, pH and other conditions to be provided for the individual processes needed, without affecting others. This increases the overall efficiency of the cell to make it compatible with life. For example, lysozomes need to degrade material using enzymes that could be harmful if they diffused around the cell globally, but by keeping them in a compartment, this process can occur whilst other organelles work. Compartmentalisation also allows for localisation of organelles that need to work together. For example, the nucleus being near the rough endoplasmic reticulum. This overall efficiency is the broad point and using specific examples of conditions and environments needed for organelles can show a good and thorough understanding of subcellular structures and how they work in a way to achieve a rate that is compatible with life.

A **poor applicant** may hear the term "cellular compartmentalisation" and begin a rehearsed spiel about what it is and how it is achieved. This is not what the question actually asks, and therefore does not really address the subject. An applicant with a poor understanding of the structure of cells may start talking about groups of cells working together as opposed to the compartments within cells. Again, this highlights gaps in fundamental concepts encountered in Biology, and suggests the applicant learns via memorisation rather than understanding what they encounter.

Q135: How true is it to say that the modern meal is the culmination of a long journey away from biology?

This is a far cry from an exam-style factual recall question and there are many angles to approach it from. It assesses many aspects of theory including digestion and evolution, but tests the applicant's ability to synthesise the facts they have learnt into a coherent argument. When thinking about the wording of "how true is it to say" it can allow you to give reasons for both sides of the statement (for and against) and there is no need to immediately polarise an answer, especially if you have not thought about this topic before.

A **good applicant** will come up with a logical approach for how to deal with this broad question. They might start by defining what the "modern meal" is – relevant terms may include; large portions, highly processed, densely caloric, high in saturated fats, fast and convenient. They could then think about the biology of eating and how this may be different for each of the factors. For example, as hunter-gatherers we were very well adapted to having a large meal and then storing excess nutrients in the form of fat in adipose tissue. This meant that we had an energy supply for respiration during periods where food was scarce. However, the modern meal is often fast and convenient which means (for many) there is never a period of scarcity and thus the excess of adipose keeps building up. In this way, the fast and convenient nature of eating whenever we feel like it has come a long way from our biology. You can also draw on increasing rates of diseases such as; obesity, diabetes and cardiovascular diseases to help illustrate points that show our body's biology is not as well adapted to the modern meal, and it is contributing to pathology and dysfunction.

A **poor applicant** may not understand the timescale at which adaptation and natural selection occurs and may talk about how we "constantly" evolve to adapt to the modern meal. Whilst evolution is a "constant" process, it happens over many generations and many years whereas the modern meal is a relatively new phenomenon that has not had enough time to cause a tangible change in human biology.

Q136: What are the effects of cocaine on cerebral and coronary blood flow?

It is unlikely this has been covered in great depth during an applicant's lessons in school so this question follows a common theme in Oxbridge-style interview questions of pushing basic concepts (in this case factors affecting blood flow) into new scenarios. The advantage of this is it means you cannot simply recall facts, but instead have to prove you have proactively engaged with them and understood them to be able to apply them into a context you will not have encountered.

A **good applicant** might not know how cocaine affects blood flow, but could go through various factors that determine flow and then address potential effects on each of these. This type of approach helps structure your thoughts and the answer you give and ensures broader coverage of the many possible effects of cocaine, even if the actual answer is not known. Blood flow can be affected by factors including; vessel diameter, turbulent or laminar blood flow, thrombus formation, viscosity of the blood itself, and pressure of the blood. By working through these factors systematically, you can hypothesise about the effects of cocaine but also demonstrate you have a secure foundation about the circulatory system and blood flow, which is more important for the interviewer to assess. In fact, cocaine is a well-known "vasoconstrictor" and it narrows the diameter of blood vessels. If after going through various factors the interviewer gives this fact to you, taking this step-by-step you can reason that cocaine therefore reduces cerebral and coronary blood flow.

This may lead onto a discussion of longer-term consequences of this blood flow and can be split into conditions that affect the brain and the heart. The key processes to consider are "hypoxia" and "ischaemia", which you will have encountered in school. A good applicant will be aware that hypoxia is a deficiency in the amount of oxygen reaching tissues but ischaemia is when inadequate blood supply results in the death of the tissue. Therefore, ischaemia is likely to be a longer-term consequence of reduced blood flow causing stroke (brain) and myocardial infarction (heart).

A **poor applicant** may not know the answer and say they have not covered this in lessons yet so cannot be sure. Even if not covered in this context, the applicant will have been taught about some of the factors affecting blood flow (for example, in the context of atherosclerosis and coronary artery disease) so should be able to attempt a response. Additionally, the applicant may simply state it "reduces it" but not go into more detail about why. Even if this is factually correct, it is less impressive for an interviewer to hear as it does not show a mechanistic understanding of blood flow and how it can be reduced/increased.

Q137: Which is better adapted- a human or a chimpanzee?

This tests understanding of the topics of evolution and adaption which are commonly encountered throughout GCSE and A-level Biology. To answer the question, you need to understand the gist of the basic process of adaptation. This is that random genetic mutations occur when organisms reproduce and the environment puts a selective pressure on a species which means that over generations more "beneficial" mutations become prevalent in the population (because they confer the selective advantage to survival, mate and reproduce) and over many generations this causes adaptation and evolution.

However, this question importantly tests the skill of being able to put forward a cogent argument; in other words, to come up with good reasons to support a point of view and present them in a coherent manner. This question also gives plenty of scope for the interviewer to "argue back" and see if the applicant can think on the spot and come up with counter arguments or spot flaws in the opposing argument. It may also lead the applicant into having to play devil's advocate and argue creatively against their original points. Therefore, it is crucial to be able to convey supporting reasons clearly and logically to support a point of view in this type of question.

A **good applicant** will understand what it means to be adapted to an environment and will then need to define 'environment', for example as the modern civilised world we live in for humans and as a jungle for chimpanzees. The argument for humans being better adapted is clearly easier and so this would be a logical point to start with. The applicant does not need to go into the ins and outs of chimpanzee biology but simple points of comparison such as bipedalism in humans allowing us to "hold" things. Being more manually dexterous could be argued as a useful adaption in our current world of machines and technology compared with brute strength which is not as necessary as it once was. Another basic point to think about is our greatly advanced level of communication.

A **poor applicant** might not understand what it means to be adapted and may simply talk about how a chimpanzee would probably win in a physical fight so they are stronger and better adapted. This argument does not make sense in relation to the question asked, but also neglects to consider that part of human adaption is our manual dexterity and ability to fashion tools (and guns) which could be used. Another poor answer could be that "humans came later so they are better adapted". This shows a poor understanding of evolution - humans and chimpanzees both evolved differently from the same ancestor around 6-8 million years ago, and whilst it is not necessary to know this exact fact, awareness of the common ancestor and how they have adapted will deter from false answers such as this.

Another sign of a poor applicant would be an inability to adapt their argument or engage in a discussion with the interviewer about why certain points they make may be less valid. This question does not solely seek to test a right or wrong initial answer but can also be used to test analytical thinking and debating skills brought out in applicants.

Q138: What is the best way to tackle the obesity epidemic?

There is no straightforward answer to this and indeed if there was, there would likely be no epidemic! This question tests your ability to come up with a logical strategy and respond effectively to counter-arguments and further probing by the interviewer. The topic of the obesity epidemic is a current issue in healthcare and medical applicants should be quite familiar with the problems faced (increasing rates of obesity in the general population as well as an alarmingly increasing rate of childhood obesity) in addition to the consequences and large strain it puts on the NHS. If it is sensible, the answer itself is less important than being able to engage in an intellectual debate about pros and cons of a given approach. Additionally, it would be a great opportunity to bring in any examples of wider reading or policies you have read about in the news (for example taxes such as the sugar tax) and discuss how they hold up against the answer selected.

A **good applicant** will show an awareness of the importance of the current obesity epidemic and suggest a sensible way to tackle it – this answer can be via a multi-faceted approach split into short-term and long-term solutions. It is important to address the cause of the epidemic, instead of purely superficial solutions. Education of the consequences of obesity and public health awareness are always solid approaches to take with such issues and you can argue that they preserve autonomy and allow a more "long-term" solution that addresses the root of the problem and has the ability to act as a preventative measure. By analytically explaining *why* the approach selected is the best way (by comparing to other alternative strategies) you can effectively answer this question. A good applicant will also be to recognise counter-arguments the interviewer may put forward and either acknowledge their validity whilst explaining why their suggested approach is better, or be flexible and try and incorporate it into their answer.

A **poor applicant** may be largely ignorant about the obesity epidemic and not be able to appreciate why it needs serious consideration. They may also suggest economically impractical solutions such as "free healthy food and exercise machines for everyone" which does not show an awareness of how healthcare systems work. Additionally, a poor applicant may only focus on "further down the line" solutions such as bariatric surgery, without addressing any form of tackling the root cause.

Q139: How would you stop the spread of Ebola if you were in charge?

This question tests your understanding of disease epidemiology and how healthcare works on the level of a population. Clearly any medical applicant who has kept up to date with the news will be able to suggest some interventions for a pandemic (in relation to COVID-19). The Ebola outbreak occurred in 2014 to 2016 in West Africa, and spread to Liberia and Sierra Leone, with scattered cases in Nigeria, Mali, Senegal, Spain, the UK, and the US. It was caused by a virus and thus many of the interventions used in COVID-19 will be translatable, however this answer will require some adaptation to acknowledge the different pattern of spread and properties of the Ebola virus. The interviewer can use this question to assess whether the applicant can suggest a variety of different measures that act in different ways, and can structure their thoughts clearly. It will also be important to be able to defend ideas and discuss them with the interviewer, who may probe further into certain approaches opted for.

A **good applicant** will have an awareness that the Ebola outbreak was caused by a virus and will tailor their answer accordingly. For a clear structure, they may split the answer into: controlling current cases, curative measures and long-term preventative control. In terms of current cases, sensible suggestions include: quarantining measures, contact tracing, PPE allocation and closing borders with neighbouring countries and of those where outbreaks are widespread. For curative measures, they may suggest funding research into potential symptomatic treatment and vaccines. In terms of preventative measures, they may suggest education and widespread public health awareness campaigns promoting good sanitation and measures to avoid zoonotic transmissions. A good candidate will also acknowledge potentially economic difficulties in implementing measures in less economically developed countries, and suggest ways around this. Additionally, a good applicant will be able to discuss why these measures are good; they tackle *both* the short-term and long-term spread of Ebola.

A **poor applicant** may have very little awareness of the Ebola outbreak and may suggest inappropriate measures for controlling a viral outbreak, for example the administration of antibiotics. A poor applicant may also suggest economically unviable approaches such as building Ebola-only hospitals across Western Africa to treat Ebola cases. Furthermore, when probed further they will likely be unable to defend their ideas or be uncomfortable going through advantages and disadvantages of their elected approaches; it is important to be able to have a discussion-style rapport with interviewers with these questions instead of expecting to present a lengthy answer and have no follow-up.

Q140: How much of human behaviour is genetically determined?

Human behaviour (innate and learned) is a topic that is often touched upon in Biology, but this question assesses an applicant's broader understanding of how complex gene-environment interactions can be. It gives the interviewer the chance to introduce more complex topics that have not been taught yet, such as epigenetics, and assess how applicants handle new information and how they adapt their answers or opinions to accommodate the new information. Therefore, to answer this question well, applicants must consider their answer in terms of a spectrum of "how much" instead of polarising their answer into simplistic terms of whether genes do or do not play a role.

A **good applicant** will give the obvious answers of behaviours that are not genetically determined (for example learning based on the environment). Learning is clearly in response to cues from the environment and different behaviours will arise from different environmental conditions. However, the applicant will realise that this is an oversimplification and that genes may have a role in predisposing certain behaviours. A common example used is the dopamine D4 receptor gene and its various polymorphisms which have been linked to behaviours such as addiction and risk-taking. Clearly there needs to be an environmental role to trigger this, but research suggests that genes can predispose an individual to be more likely to display certain behaviours. Other examples can be genetic factors involved in some psychiatric conditions including schizophrenia. If introduced to the concept of epigenetics (the environment affecting how genes are expressed), a good applicant will be able to adapt their initial estimate of how much behaviour is genetically determined and explain this to the interviewer. The use of examples is key to answering questions such as these in a tangible way and to avoid being vague.

A good applicant may also be asked how they would set up an experiment to investigate this question. Like with previous questions, it is important you realise that you will likely have to work through your answer with the interviewer and not get phased about the prospect of having to present a flawless answer on the first pass.

A **poor applicant** may not listen to the question carefully and talk about nature versus nurture in a broader sense without referring to behaviour specifically. This is likely to be a more comfortable topic for applicants to talk about as they can mention clear examples of genetically determined traits such as eye colour. However, it is important to select which examples to use carefully, and to only consider those that relate to behaviour, as the question is not designed to have a clear cut answer and should involve some profound thinking.

Q141: Why is sustainability so difficult to achieve?

This is a very broad question and an applicant can approach barriers to sustainability from many angles (economic and financial, innovational, social, political, institutional to name a few). In contrast to some of the more factual types, this question allows the interviewer to see how creative you can be in thinking about challenges towards this goal and may result in the interviewer trying to push you to think of difficulties beyond the commonly given reasons. It may also be a platform for the interviewer to then ask you to think of ways to solve the aforementioned difficulties. Therefore, it is important for you to approach this question with as open a mind as possible and to remember to think on the spot and not always with a formulaic approach of pre-rehearsed facts.

A **good applicant** might briefly begin by defining their understanding of sustainability. This checks they are thinking along the right tracks but also buys some time to think. A good definition might be the ability to meet the needs of the current population without compromising those of the future. Some intrinsic social difficulties that arise from this definition are that the needs themselves are on the rise with a rapidly growing population. A good applicant may also talk about some of the barriers to sustainability in an economic sense (often the sustainable source of a product or energy is more expensive and profit is often prioritised). When thinking about it from a research point of view there are barriers in terms of innovation and knowledge, such as the obstacles to nuclear fusion (a topic covered at GCSE Physics). By looking at the issue from different fields, you can show creativity and breadth but must be prepared to be asked about one or two of these in further depth.

A **poor applicant** may be phased by the lack of rehearsal for this type of question, which does not tackle some of the typical human Biology expected at a medical interview. They may be unwilling to think about the difficulties from multiple angles and only talk about the population growing and demanding more resources. A poor applicant may vaguely talk about fossil fuels running out but be unable to explicitly link this to the question – that we have a reliance on non-renewable sources of energy, possibly for economic reasons and their finite nature makes them unsustainable.

Q142: What are the dangers of an ageing population? Is ageing a disease?

The first question allows an interviewer to assess how aware the applicant is about current challenges faced by healthcare systems, whereas the second question leaves more room for the applicant to be assessed on creativity and the ability to formulate arguments on both sides of a point of view. The concept of an ageing population is commonly encountered, from a medical perspective, relating to future strains on public healthcare and most applicants will have come across this. The second question has come up in a similar form as a past BMAT essay question, and allows the interviewer to assess how well the applicant understands what a disease is and the difference between quality of life and quantity of life. This will help distinguish those applicants who have a genuine interest in the vocation, and have been doing some cursory thinking and reading about the roles and challenges of a doctor and the move in healthcare away from extending life purely for the sake of years.

A **good applicant** will be able to engage with the first question and suggest multiple dangers of an ageing population, including the strain this can place on a healthcare system as elderly people tend to have more co-morbidities and need complex care. A good applicant will be able to give a sensible definition of disease and talk about arguments both for and against ageing being a disease, whilst giving their own personal opinion. When thinking of ageing as a disease, you could mention age-related diseases and complications (for example, osteoporosis). When thinking about why ageing is not a disease, you should be able to allude to the fact that ageing is a natural process and there is a strong argument against trying to instinctively fight it. A good applicant may even be able to link the second question to wider reading they have done, such as a popular book by Atul Gawande called 'Being Mortal' which looks at end-of-life care and the idea that medicine should seek to promote well-being rather than simply seeking to make patients survive as long as possible.

A **poor applicant** may misunderstand what an ageing population is (growth in the proportion and number of older persons in the population) and may simply talk about the dangers of ageing for the first question. In approaching the second question, a poor applicant may have a superficial understanding of disease and simply answer "yes ageing is a disease as it makes you less healthy" without even appreciating arguments for the other side. When asked a more subjective question, applicants should strive to think about the arguments on each side as part of their "thinking out loud" before analytically explaining why they have arrived at a point of view.

Q143: Do we actually need a brain?

This question assesses how well an applicant can engage with a seemingly simple question and can give them a chance to show creativity and lateral thinking on a backdrop of simple Biology. To answer this question effectively you need to creatively come up with different "levels" at which to answer this. For example, you could talk about: whether we need a brain to live versus to think versus to perform other functions etc., or whether there are alternative structures. You could even consider if we need a whole brain or only part of it. By engaging with this question, the interviewer can see how well an applicant can think laterally and use their imagination to look at a question in a fresh way and come up with interesting answers.

The mark of a **good applicant** will be the ability to structure their thoughts and vocalise their thought process. For an unrehearsed question, this can seem intimidating, but it is useful for the interviewer to hear the applicant's thought process instead of having an applicant sit in silence for a few minutes before making a point. You could approach it by thinking about what the brain does, and think whether these functions are vital to life or could be replaced by other mechanisms. By splitting "need" into survival or higher function paves the way into arguments revolving around the need for the brain stem versus the rest of the brain. For interest, "Mike the headless chicken" is a good example for thinking about the value of the brainstem. A good applicant may also try and think of examples where people have survived with compromised brain function (for example, tumours, injuries) and use this as a stepping stone for thoughts about whether we need the whole brain as we know it, or only certain areas.

A **poor applicant** might be unwilling to engage with this question creatively, and may simply answer it on a superficial level. They will likely say "yes of course, we need our brains to survive" but then be unwilling to extend their reasoning beyond this. Upon probing, or hints from the interviewer to think about what we actually use our brains for, the applicant may reveal shaky foundations of knowledge and give answers such as "we use it to think every day" without applying knowledge from their GCSEs and A-levels about specific areas of the brain they have encountered, such as the hypothalamus, the pituitary gland or the cerebellum. As is often the case, this delineates between those who have understood and questioned the concepts taught to them and those who have accepted facts passively.

Q144: What does the kidney do?

The kidney is a big topic covered in Biology both in GCSE and A-level, and this question provides a starting point for the interviewer to assess how well an applicant understands the topic and whether they have simply committed some facts to memory or have understood core principles that will be built upon in medical school. The interviewer can use this broad question as a springboard to go in various directions; asking more about one function in particular to a higher level or perhaps by asking why the kidney is well placed to perform the functions mentioned.

A **good applicant** will answer this question in a structured manner, by listing some key functions of the kidneys as an "overview" and then going into some of them in more depth as needed. When answering a question such as this, it is important not to "brain dump" everything you know about the kidneys such as the anatomy and structure, but instead keep everything relevant to the question at hand, i.e. their *function*. Some key functions to mention are excretion of wastes and toxins, regulation of ion concentration (and pH) and regulation of osmolarity and extracellular fluid production. Some lesser-known functions include the production of hormones (for example, renin). A good applicant should be prepared to be stretched, for example the interviewer may talk about a disease that affects the kidney in a certain way and ask how the body will be affected. By understanding the core functions of the kidney, you will be able to make guesses as to what will happen when this regulatory role goes awry and start extending yourself into the type of thinking needed at medical school.

A **poor applicant** may see this as a chance to go through everything they know about the kidneys in great detail to show off their factual recall. In fact, the question concerns the function of the kidneys and the applicant should make sure to keep the discussion focussed around this and keep returning to the question posed. Additionally, a poor applicant may run into issues if they can recall the functions factually without a deeper understanding of how this occurs. When further probed, they may find it harder to hypothesise what may happen to the body when this function is compromised or when a similar follow-up question is asked. It is always important to make sure the applicant understands key topics taught at school and is not simply regurgitating facts.

Q145: Why does our heart beat faster when we exercise?

This is a key concept covered in Biology and applicants should be able to engage with this with knowledge they have already encountered in their lessons so far. However, this question also tackles key concepts covered in Physiology at medical school and allows the interviewer to try and "push" the applicant out of their comfort zone and engage with material similar to that in the first few years of medical school. Most Oxbridge interviews indeed mimic the supervision set-up at medical school where the supervisor teaches concepts or pushes students, and therefore this can be a chance to assess how well an applicant thrives in this style of learning. Therefore, when answering this type of question you should begin with the fundamentals you do know but not be afraid if the interviewer starts introducing graphs or new equations and you should try engage with it as actively as you can to demonstrate that you are teachable.

A **good applicant** will have a robust understanding of the basics of the cardiovascular system as taught at GCSE and A-level. They will explain what happens logically starting from the fact that when we exercise, parts of our bodies like the skeletal muscles need more oxygen and they also create waste products at a faster rate which need to be removed. This happens via blood flow, and the applicant may go into some detail about how red blood cells achieve this. They will then remember the question asks for why the heart must beat faster and link this to the state which exercise induces. The heart is the pump that ensures the blood circulates around your body, by beating faster it can meet the increased needs of the body that occur when we exercise. This may lead to some discussion about cardiac output (the rate at which blood is pumped out of the heart) and how heart rate forms a part of this, as well as stroke volume (the volume of blood ejected by the heart with each beat). Regardless of the direction it takes, a good applicant will understand the basics of the question and will be willing to stretch their learning as the interviewer sees fit.

A **poor applicant** may have a superficial understanding of the heart as a pump and not realise that this must adapt to meet the needs of the body. This will clearly hinder their ability to respond to this question, and will help the interviewer assess which applicants understand the content they are being taught, and which applicants simply memorise a collection of facts such as the definition of the heart. Additionally, poor applicants may be unwilling to push themselves with new concepts introduced by the interviewer and only want to discuss things they know for sure, which shows signs that a supervision-style of teaching does not work well for them.

Q146: What else do doctors do apart from treating patients?

This question assesses how aware applicants are about what a career in medicine entails, and how realistic their expectations of the job are. Work experience, speaking to doctors and background research on the internet can all be used to inform this answer and can help you demonstrate that you have taken the decision to pursue medicine seriously. An interviewer can use this to differentiate between applicants who are serious about the vocation from those who have simply applied to the course due to having "good grades" and seeing hyperbolised media representations of the job.

A **good applicant** will be aware of the fact that within the role of "practitioner" there are many duties including a large amount of administrative work and other roles such as comforting the relatives of a patient in some cases. A good applicant will have likely read some of the GMC's guidelines about the duties and roles of a doctor and will also make reference to other roles a doctor can be involved in such as the "scientist" aspect and the "teacher". For Oxbridge in particular, the "scientist" role of a doctor is not to be neglected as the compulsory intercalation year clearly requires you to have an interest in at least considering academic components of the job. Additionally, anyone who has undertaken clinical experience will not be able to avoid seeing a "teaching" role of a doctor. This can happen in a variety of ways and some doctors are more formally and actively involved in teaching than others, but it is almost certain that at some point in their career, a doctor will be involved in teaching someone more junior.

A **poor applicant** may not have put in much effort to researching what it means to be a doctor and may have simply based their expectations from shows on TV/other dramatic media representations. This question can clearly vet for this and a poor applicant may struggle to suggest any other roles of a doctor. Especially during COVID-19, it is not compulsory to have undertaken clinical work experience and observed the roles of a doctor first-hand, but with the information available on the internet, there is no real excuse for not having some answer to this question.

Q147: If you have the money to do either 1 heart transplant or 100 hip replacements? Which one would you do and why?

This question is assessing an applicant's approach to medical ethics and the issues surrounding limited resources and their allocation. It is clear that there is no obvious answer, and this question will involve weighing up both sides and being able to come to a conclusion and defend why you picked it, whilst acknowledging the valid points for the other option. In terms of medical ethics, this question can assess how much background reading you have done around this common type of scenario - there is definitely no expectation to be an expert in the field, but some mention of utilitarianism, the pillar of justice or other key concepts will help show an interviewer you have engaged with this side of medicine. For interest, QALY is a good way to approach these types of health intervention questions. Another skill this question will test is the ability for an applicant to formulate arguments analytically and have a debate about the two options – the interviewer will likely take an opposing stance regardless of the outcome you pick, and this will test your ability to think on their feet.

A **good applicant** will weigh up both sides out loud but then explain why they have picked the option they go for. For the heart transplant, you can talk about how if this is successful, it will undoubtedly help save a person's life as a transplant is often used as a last resort when other options have failed. They could mention points about how it could be used to save a person who has their whole life ahead of them and so might compare with regards to QALY to the hip replacements option. An obvious argument for the side of the hip replacements is the utilitarian approach of pleasing the most people, which is a branch of consequentialism. However, it should be acknowledged that a hip replacement is typically only used in people who will gain less years of life after the surgery as it tends to be needed in older patients and is also not "life-saving" in the way a heart transplant is. By weighing out these pros and cons out loud, you will buy some time to come to an answer but also show a thorough understanding of some of the ethical arguments behind this scenario. You should eventually pick one of the outcomes (for example, the hip replacements) and be able to validate why you have opted for this – restoring mobility to 100 people would be a great outcome from the utilitarian point of view versus saving the life of 1 person with a risky surgery.

A **poor applicant** might only state advantages for the side they pick without acknowledging any of the arguments for the other option. It is important to realise that in an ideal world with enough resources you would be able to offer all 101 surgeries, and there is no need to convince the interviewer otherwise (for example by saying "hip replacements are not even that important" if trying to argue for the heart transplant). It is much better to sensitively show that you understand the validity of both options but to come to a well-reasoned conclusion. A poor applicant may also fail to come to a conclusion and be unable to pick a side – this does not allow the interviewer to assess their ability to debate or argue analytically and will not be very helpful for testing the skills associated with this.

Q148: Discuss the ethical dilemma of Huntingdon's disease when one family member knows they have it and don't want anyone else to know.

This question tests your awareness of medical ethics and some of the basic tenets of professionalism, as described by the General Medical Council (GMC). Discussion of medical ethics allows an interviewer to see if you can see multiple points of view and it is always important to discuss arguments on either side of the situation at hand. It also provides a springboard for the interviewer to play devil's advocate and ask you to justify your views in the face of opposing arguments. Therefore, with questions such as these, the answer itself is just as important as the way it is conveyed and discussed. Importantly, if the applicant is not aware of Huntingdon's disease, it is better to ask or clarify specifics (that it is an inherited neurodegenerative disease with an autosomal dominant pattern) - it is a disease often covered in the genetics topics of Biology, but if the applicant is not aware of it they are better placed to ask the interviewer and make sure they are forming arguments for the right dilemma, than to miss key arguments due to not understanding the issue of it having a genetic inheritance pattern.

A **good applicant** will be aware that Huntingdon's has an autosomal dominant pattern of inheritance, and thus if one person has the mutation, it is highly likely others have it and it has not arisen spontaneously. A good applicant will *discuss* the dilemma by paying attention to the arguments on both sides, making sure not to be purely one-sided in their approach. The pillar of autonomy and confidentiality can be used to explain why an individual may not want family members to know and, for example, treat them differently. However, the genetic nature of the disease means that by not telling their family they do not give other members a chance to understand their own personal risks of the disease and obtain genetic testing, or even have enough time to mentally prepare for the complications if found to be positive for the mutation. It is also something that a potential partner of this person should be aware of before deciding whether to have children who are genetically related versus adoption. The key to answering this question is discussing both sides and being able to acknowledge and state all arguments, even if the applicant personally falls very strongly on one side.

A **poor applicant** may have no understanding of the genetic element of the disease and will not try to clarify this before launching into arguments about confidentiality being the most important thing to consider and that the family has no right to know. Additionally, a poor applicant may be purely one-sided in their answer. When given an ethical dilemma at interview, there will often be arguments that should be considered for both sides and the applicant must always make sure they push aside personal beliefs and at least state one argument for each side to show they have the analytical ability to recognise the "dilemma".

Q149: Will 3D printing revolutionise medicine?

You can have fun with this question! How you approach it is up to you – there are many different angles of attack and it depends on your interests. This is a really nice opportunity to show off some knowledge about whatever you have been reading about that you think might be part of the medical revolution. You have to first answer the question, by evaluating the role of 3D printing in medicine and what its uses may be. Any knowledge on how it has already been used in medicine shows you are keeping up to date with current events and demonstrates enthusiasm in the field. Think about situations in which current practice would *change* if there were 3D printing opportunities - this is what revolutionises means. You don't want to just give examples of where it is useful now, this doesn't fully answer the question. You might also want to consider the limitations of 3D printing (remember you always want to have a semblance of a balanced argument!).

Once you have addressed the question, if you have another particular interest that you think will revolutionise medicine *more*, now is your time to shine. If you think gene therapy or AI is the key to changing the landscape of medicine, tell the interviewers! Just remember to conclude by summarising your arguments and addressing the question one last time (much like a BMAT essay).

Good applicant: 3D printing technology has already been used for various purposes in education and surgery. It has been used for recreating models for training purposes e.g., for emergency procedures like cricothyroidotomies, as well as for surgeons to practice on before an actual surgery. This has particular potential to revolutionise surgical oncology, where specific tumours can be recreated from scans and help surgeons better visualise the anatomy – potentially making it possible to effectively perform surgery on previously inoperable tumours. 3D printing has also been used as a much cheaper and faster way to make prosthetics, which again can be tailored to be patient-specific and increasing functionality. Finally in surgery, bespoke single-use instruments can be made (much cheaper than normal ways of manufacturing), which might help open up the realm of what is currently possible in microscopic and laparoscopic surgery. I think where 3D printing has the most potential is in bioprinting, where it has been used to print layers of living tissue to form organoids which are being used for research purposes. Organoids give us an understanding of how cells work together to make functioning tissues and how tissues come together in structure and function to create an organ and will give us a huge amount of insight into both the physiology and pathology of organs, as well as the effect of drugs/treatments. They have already been used for skin grafting, but as the technology advances could also be used for organ transplants. If this potential is realised, I think it could really revolutionise medicine because it would firstly address the organ crisis, but also help cure diseases that result from organ dysfunction such as type I diabetes.

Note, the author of this answer does believe in the power of 3D printing but one does not have to agree with this, and could argue that something else is equally if not more important in the future of medicine.

A bad applicant would simply list the uses of 3D printing without addressing why it might be good for medicine and demonstrating an understanding of how the field could change as a result of popularisation of 3D printing.

PSYCHOLOGY

Applicants from a range of backgrounds may be asked questions on psychology, experiment design or statistics and data-handling. The interviewers understand that some applicants may not have studied psychology before – be prepared to address unexpected questions, and show through extra-curricular reading or activities how you've fostered broad interests.

The questions below are specific to psychology, but **there is no guarantee that 'psychology' questions will be asked** in a bio science interview. Be prepared to answer questions that are open-ended, require some knowledge of popular psychology topics (e.g. well-known psychiatric conditions), require you to design experiments or metrics, and that show you can use statistical or other objective approaches to answer subjective questions. Remember that **neuroscience is a part of psychology**, so you may be asked about cognitive functions or sensory systems.

WORKED QUESTIONS

Below are a few examples of how to start breaking down an interview question, complete with model answers.

Q1: What do you know about learning in infants?

There are a number of different ways this question could develop, and it is open-ended enough that it is possible to steer towards areas of particular knowledge or interest. Taking a neurological approach could mean discussing neuronal mechanisms involved with learning and memory (e.g. forging new synapse connections). It could also involve discussions of cognitive pathways, for instance, the functioning of normal versus impaired language centres in the cortex, and language acquisition.

Taking a psychological approach could involve discussing <u>normal human developmental milestones and Piaget's learning stages</u>. It could also involve a discussion of different types of conditioning (e.g. Pavlov), and how feedback from consequences and rewards influence behaviour. A social psychological discussion may include how individuals take cues from parents and society to learn (though remember the question specifies babies). This is also a chance to discuss any recent research encountered. For instance, a new study showing that mother rats lastingly pass down their specific fears to their babies through the scents they emit when reacting to specific triggers.

Q2: How would you go about measuring intelligence?

This is a question about metrics and there are several ways you could start this answer off. You could <u>define intelligence</u> in any way you like, and then set up some systems for measuring that definition of intelligence, or you could start by discussing the concept of intelligence and suggest some ways to constrain both the definition and level of intelligence simultaneously. For instance, you could define intelligence as a set of mental abilities, such as logic, spatial awareness, numeracy and memory, and suggest tests of each ability. Or you could mention current intelligence metrics and discuss which abilities they measure and ignore, whether they are representing different societal ideas about intelligence and intelligent figures, and if they work cross-culturally and through time.

For example, using IQ testing as a starting point, you could discuss the different types of questions it presents and which people will score high and low (e.g. spatial questions can be a large component of some versions of the test and men often have better spatial reasoning skills). You could discuss some of its advantages (e.g. that it scores on a bell curve with 100 at the centre to normalise a sample of test-takers) and disadvantages (e.g. that it is not an absolute scoring system so comparisons may be false). You could discuss related effects, such as the <u>Flynn Effect</u> (apparent rising of IQ over time as modern test-takers score above average on older IQ tests), and whether these work in the favour of these tests as valid metrics.

Remember that however you argue, you are not setting out to defend a personal viewpoint, but are discussing the strengths and weaknesses of a number of definitions and metrics from different perspectives, including recognising those ways of thinking which may be Western-centric.

Q3: Are diseases like schizophrenia caused more by nature or nurture?

This is a classic nature-nurture question with a psychology twist. A good way to start this question is to define nature and nurture as the genes inherited from parents and the environment exposed to during development. At this point you can showcase some knowledge of schizophrenia; you could perhaps cite the rates of incidence in relatives of schizophrenics versus the general population, or some adoption studies monitoring the incidence of the disease in children raised by their schizophrenic parent or by unaffected adoptive parents. If you have no knowledge of schizophrenia, you could ask if you can generalise the question to similar psychiatric disorders.

To continue, you might want to discuss the different ways you could be affected by nature and nurture. For instance, you could inherit genes that directly predispose you to schizophrenia or to conditions which make you vulnerable to schizophrenia, such as a related condition or a neurotransmitter imbalance, etc. You could also be epigenetically affected through the impact of schizophrenia on lifestyle, for instance, leading to damaged DNA in gametes or the transmission of phobias and anxieties in DNA, as has been shown possible in some recent studies. For nurture, you might want to mention in vivo effects of drugs and alcohol or stress and poor nutrition on a developing baby. Also after birth, the effects of having an ill parent, such as poor care or trauma as an infant, learning bad habits by imitation or other conditioning to an unhealthy mental state. Or having a generally bad childhood potentially leaving an individual more disposed to psychiatric conditions. The important part of this question is breaking down the effects of nature and nurture in a thorough discussion, rather than demonstrating perfect knowledge of schizophrenia.

Q4: Can you define synaesthesia? What is its importance?

The first part of this question would allow you to show that you have taken an interest in psychology, particularly if you haven't studied psychology at school, and the second part would show how you reason about the brain. Synaesthesia is a famous neurological abnormality where <u>stimulation of one sensory or cognitive pathway leads to the automatic stimulation of another</u>, particularly one not usually associated with the first. For instance, the letter 'S' may always seem red or the number 'I' may sound like the note middle C. Synaesthesia is a favourite of the popular neuroscientist, V.S. Ramachandran. If you haven't heard of synaesthesia, say so, you can still answer the second part of the question. Synaesthesia is thought to be caused by <u>cross-activation of brain regions</u>, so the most common forms hint at which brain regions are adjacent. This can then be used for cortex mapping. It also may hint at which cognitions and sensory concepts are processed in similar ways, as the prevalence of some forms and directions of synaesthesia over others may suggest that those cognitions and sensory concepts are encoded similarly in the brain.

Q5: How can we identify our 'known unknowns'?

This question is designed to push you to think in the abstract; to show that you can work on a problem where all definitive answers are off the table and to see what unique thoughts you can have. Any approach to this question will be individual and rely on your ability to think originally. Some ideas you might want to consider in your answer, if you are stuck, are: distinguishing between individual and societal knowledge (e.g. knowing what you don't know by comparing to other members of society), or specific instances of <u>definable ignorance versus an overall lack of knowledge</u> (e.g. not knowing someone's phone number versus not knowing there is a great concept in our understanding of physics completely untouched, such as quantum mechanics in the 19th century). You could also take a neurological approach, discussing how the brain fills in gaps in knowledge automatically to reconcile reality to what the brain 'knows', perhaps citing an instance where this malfunctions and renders a situation unknowable.

For instance, in anosognosia, where, for example, people suffering from a paralysed limb believe that they are not paralysed due to a failure in reconciling the dissonance between the command to move a paralysed limb and the visual feedback that no movement is occurring. Whatever the approach to this question, it is important to show an understanding of the <u>different types of knowledge</u> and the different ways we can understand knowledge, both in our own minds and academically.

Q6: Which animal would you say was the most conscious?

This question is clearly aiming at consciousness and our understanding of it, which is known to be the 'hard question' of psychology. It is important to define whether by 'animal' the interviewer means only non-human animals. Should that be the case, the interviewer does not necessarily expect a 'right' or a 'wrong' answer. It is very difficult to assess whether a chimpanzee or a dolphin is 'more' conscious than the other. Indeed, it is very difficult to assess the consciousness of anyone that is not us, even our fellow human beings: the only reason we assume they are conscious is because they tell us so.

A good answer would take into account the <u>difficulties of defining consciousness</u> and assessing it in non-verbal creatures. It is also important not to get confused and equate consciousness with intelligence: there might be a good reason to believe that a monkey is 'more conscious' than a goldfish, but it is necessary to define the relationship between intelligence and consciousness and not conflate the two. Should the interviewer include humans in the question, it might be worth discussing <u>the evolutionary importance of consciousness</u>, how it may have developed in humans, and whether 'proto-consciousness can be found in animals. Again, a few sentences highlighting the difficulties of defining and assessing consciousness are needed.

Q7: Is IQ a valid measurement of intelligence?

Intelligence is a complicated construct that most people have an opinion of, which makes it difficult to discuss in psychological terms. The question seems to be aiming at two things: first, provoking a discussion on our understanding of intelligence, the many different things it can mean, and how it can mean different things to different people. For example, in some cultures, intelligence may be regarded as something different than what many people in the Western world equate with intelligence. Indeed, upon inspection, there might be a large divergence in what individuals within a culture believe intelligence to be. Some issues that may come up are whether there is one intelligence or many, whether intelligence is learned or inherited, whether intelligence can change over time. The second point the question is trying to get at, which is closely related to the previous points, is regarding the measurement of intelligence. If you know about IQ and how it is quantified, here is your opportunity to demonstrate your knowledge. Always take into consideration, however, that you have to answer the question and not get side tracked. If you do not know much about IQ, it is your opportunity to deduce what it is from an intelligent conversation: if you had to invent a way to measure intelligence, how would you do it? The interviewer will help you if you get stuck, and once you do it, try to steer back the conversation to see if the new method wholly covers what you believe is intelligence, examining what the possible pitfalls may be.

Q8: What do we mean when we discuss 'activity in the brain'?

This question is double-edged: on one hand, it is an opportunity to demonstrate your knowledge of different brain scanning techniques. If you know a little about functional magnetic resonance imaging or other methods to scan for brain activity, here you have the opportunity to demonstrate your knowledge and discuss them. If you happen to not know much about brain scanning methods at the point this question is asked, do not panic for the interviewers are more interested in how you engage with difficult issues rather than looking for any concrete knowledge that you may or may not have.

It is indeed a bit of a philosophical question: if we see brain activity in a certain brain region during a certain task, what does it really mean? In many experiments, people are told to do a certain task while their brain activity is measured, and certain inferences are made based on the outcome. For example, the amygdala has become known as the fear centre of the brain for its strong activity during fear-related stimuli. But does this tell us that amygdala activation is both necessary and sufficient for experiencing fear? The brain is an extraordinarily interconnected system, is it really possible to isolate individual parts? More importantly, is it possible to isolate psychological processes, such as fear or attention? Just because we subjectively feel that they are isolatable does not mean that they actually are.

Q9: What would you say was the ideal personality for a world leader?

This sort of question may arise as a prompt to discuss personality or as an interesting discussion point in places where students are able to study both psychology and politics. Given the priority on psychology, it would be recommended that the answer begins with a definition of personality, what it means, what people usually understand it to mean, and perhaps on how it can be measured. Once you feel you have covered your bases, it would be interesting to incorporate the answer as to what a world leader would require. World leaders, be it in business or politics, generally need to be charismatic and able to convince people to work for them. Does this mean that they have to have a highly empathetic personality? On the other hand, these leaders often have to make difficult decisions that involve considerable sacrifices. Does this mean they need a particular sort of psychopathy that helps them understand individuals but not care about them? If we assume so, how does this fit into the personality structures that exist? How would one measure this? World leaders are often (but by no means always) thought to be intelligent: is intelligence part of a personality?

Q10: Would you say that questioning users of psychedelics produces useful data on cognition?

In the early days of psychology, a lot of research was performed on subjective reports of individuals. The problem with this research was that it was difficult to verify and confirm, and was not objective due to its very nature. Psychological research then attempted to move on to more objective measures, such as behaviour, which many people believe was a very important step towards establishing the validity of psychology as a science. On the other hand, interesting psychological constructs, such as consciousness, are very difficult to experiment on objectively. Drugs are interesting because by chemically altering the way the brain works, experimenters can make deductions about how the brain works. For example, most <u>psychotropic substances alter time perception</u>, which could be used to determine whether time perception depends on a specific part of the brain, or whether it is a broader function involving several parts of the brain. In addition, if a particular substance affects both certain types of vision and certain types of movement, it could be assumed that the two are somehow linked together. That being said, there are ethical questions raised by reliance on psychotropic substances in a research setting, such as their almost ubiquitous illegality or their effect on health, which should be taken into account before research is done in this way.

Q11: What can autism show us about the way we understand others?

Autism spectrum disorder is characterised by a wide variety of cognitive and behavioural symptoms, most characteristically problems in social issues. For example, people with autism are often thought to be highly interested in routines and numbers (e.g. a train schedule) whereas they seem to show very little interest towards other human beings or other games children like to play, like role-playing games. By studying the problems that people with autism have, we can perhaps get an insight into how healthy people think about others. It is well known that people with autism have trouble <u>identifying and understanding human emotion</u> from a very early age.

This can tell us many things, perhaps the most important of which is the realisation that it is surprisingly intuitive and easy for us to perform highly complicated tasks such as understanding what other people are feeling and why. By studying the development of autistic children and identifying the errors that they make compared to the errors of healthy children, we might be able to identify the mental processes that are behind our intuitive social appraisals and understand at what point and why they start to differ.

Q12: How can we determine whether we are capable of thought?

This question can be answered in a vast variety of ways, my answer will approach it from an evolutionary psychology point of view. First of all, I would like to point out that it is possible to dispute the premise of the question: we indeed know that we think, but often we overestimate exactly how aware we are of our mental processes. Psychology researchers looking at decision-making have discovered that human beings are quite unaware of how they come to decisions and how extraneous factors, such as the irrelevant number they had been presented earlier, can affect their decisions. This is important, for one could also argue it is better to ask: "why do we think we know that we think".

Nonetheless, it is safe to assume that we do indeed have a certain degree of awareness of our own thoughts and I propose two reasons why this may have developed. First, this awareness may have developed in human beings because it helps us understand why we behave in the way we do, which facilitates complex tasks like making tools or solving problems (i.e. I am looking for sharp stones so I can make an arrow that can kill an animal which I can then eat). Secondly, humans are highly social animals and knowing why we do things may help us understand why others do things, which can provide us with a competitive advantage.

Q13: Can you reliably learn about someone's personality by asking them about it?

First of all, it is necessary to distinguish what the question means by personality. The construct of personality is defined in myriad ways, but it is generally believed to be a group of individual characteristics, usually thought to be relatively stable over time, which can be used to predict and explain behaviour. Taking that into account, most personality tests, such as the Big 5, take the approach of asking individuals a set of questions and scoring the answers in order to place the individual along different dimensions of personality or in different groups. This has some merits: the resulting values are quite stable over time (if you take the same test a week apart you get the same result), between individuals (if you take the test and a good friend takes the test answering he or she thinks you would, you can expect the results to be quite similar) and can be used to predict behaviour to a certain extent.

However, there are a few downsides to asking people questions to determine their personality. First, it <u>assumes that people are aware of what their personality is</u>. Cognitive psychological research, particularly in decision-making, has demonstrated that people are very unaware of many things we would intuitively consider to be consciously accessible information. Secondly, it assumes that people will answer accurately questions relating to personality (they may be biased to answer in a certain way or to please the person asking, or to stick to cultural norms). Other, new methods, such as those which rely on using behavioural footprints online, have recently become increasingly accurate in predicting the personality of individuals.

Q14: Do you think individuals all behave similarly in controlled situations?

This question is hinting at the person-situation debate in psychology, in which psychologists long debated whether an individual's personality or the situation is more predictive of behaviour. On one hand, influential studies like Stanley Milgram's electrocution experiments and Phillip Zimbardo's Stanford prison experiment showed that ordinary individuals are prone to act in extraordinary ways in certain circumstances, supporting the claim that the situation is more important than the person. On the other hand, as many other researchers pointed out, not even in those experiments did everyone behave in the same way, and there are various reasons to believe that the methodology of the study did not quite support the arguments made by the original researchers. For example, people who are keen to participate in a "prison experiment" are likely to be different from most people. Of course, it seems to be true that both factors matter: both the person and the situation.

Overall, different people often behave similarly in similar situations because in most cases it makes sense to do so: if we had to think explicitly about what to do every time we do something, everything we do would involve a significant amount of effort. Therefore, it makes sense to copy others or follow certain behavioural schemas in many situations, not least because it is expected from us by other people. That being said, it is fairly evident that different people do tend to behave differently in the same situation, which is perhaps evidenced by the range of different behaviours interviewers witness in the interview setting.

Q15: Why do we have auditory hallucinations, and how do they relate to schizophrenia?

What we perceive the world to be is not so much what is actually out there but rather the reality that our brain constructs out of our sensory inputs: our vision, our hearing, our tactile input, etc. This is an extraordinarily complex process as there is a lot of noise in the world and our brain is constantly engaged in separating the useful information from the less useful information, and to do so, it often makes inferences such as assuming that an unheard word was based on the context.

In some cases, these inferences are incorrect, even for healthy individuals, for example, when one wrongly thinks someone said your name. Importantly, these inferences are dependent on a considerable amount of prior beliefs such as what sort of word fits in a particular sentence or what sort of things people say.

Schizophrenics are known to sometimes have auditory hallucinations, often appearing in the form of persecutory voices. It is possible that schizophrenics hear voices that are not there because they have trouble making the correct inferences, perhaps confusing their own internal beliefs with outside stimuli. In this case, <u>auditory hallucinations might be the product of a highly effective but imperfect</u> system (hence the mistakes made by healthy individuals) which is incorrectly calibrated in the case of schizophrenia.

COURSEWORK INTERVIEWS

When applying to do Biological Natural Sciences (including Experimental Psychology) at Cambridge, or possibly Biology or Psychology at Oxford, an applicant may be asked to submit coursework and be called for a coursework interview. Usually, in the morning on the day of the interview, this work is submitted and read by the interviewer. The work is used as a basis for discussion of research and experimental methods and analysis.

The interviewer may open by asking for a summary of the piece of work, the methodology behind it, and the results obtained. They may then ask some follow-up questions related to the work or the subject matter. This part of the interview will be very individual and depend on the nature and subject of the work submitted.

After the discussion of the work, the interviewer will probably guide the conversation toward some questions about experimental methods and analysis to test the applicant's ability to think like a scientist. For example:

Q16: What experiment would you design to determine whether rats can differentiate colours?

Answering this question would involve suggesting model experiments and how to analyse the data. Perhaps the rats could be presented with <u>different coloured tiles</u>, and when they step on one of the colours they receive a treat. As the tiles are removed and replaced in new positions, the number of times the rats stepped on the food-giving colour could be counted, and this data analysed for a significant correlation. The point of these questions is to suggest different ideas and to show an understanding of their strengths and weakness and an ability to use data usefully.

Q17: Why do bats and moles have the same sized body, but different sized brains?

Those of you knowledgeable about bats may immediately think of their brain-power-demanding echolocation and it's OK to say this idea, but remember to think like a scientist and make sure you aren't jumping to conclusions. This is a chance for you to ask testable questions which may constrain the answer. Ask first: Which brain is bigger? Is the whole brain bigger or is one part, such as the cortex, disproportionately large? Then perhaps: is it that the brain is too large/small for the animal's body size or the body which is too large/small for the brain size? You might then use specific knowledge of the mole (e.g. lives in dark) and bat (flies) life-habit, and of brain function in relation to size to give all of the possible justified answers to these questions, and maybe <u>design simple tests to rule out certain answers or favour others</u>.

Q18: What do you expect to get out of this degree?

This has to be a truthful answer, as with any of these 'generic' questions. The interviewer will have heard every conceivable answer before, so you need to explain your personal reasoning, rather than tuning your answer to what you think the interviewer wants to hear. However, it is always beneficial in these types of questions to have at least one element that you deem unique (or as close as you can get) to you. The more personality you can bring to your answer, especially the unique element, the better it will likely be received.

This could be a warm-up question, or it may be used as a finishing question after some technical assessments. If the former, you can include potential technical challenges/processes from your prospective degree, for example if you are aware that there will be essay writing or scientific paper writing. If the latter, it would be great if you could refer back to the technical assessments from the interview in some way. For example, if you were interpreting graphs and reporting data findings in one technical assessment, a great answer would incorporate that (providing it has a degree of truth of course):

"I really enjoy exploring data and interpreting findings, but it is something I have limited exposure to in school. I'd love to engage with the research fellows in my faculty, to better understand how they do this when reviewing and publishing studies, so that I can better my skills."

Notice how this answer refers to research fellows, an aspect of university and Oxbridge value very highly. Your recognition of what you have done, combined with your engagement with this aspect of your prospective degree, will sound very appesing to a tutor.

A good answer to this question will incorporate the above, alongside one or two generic points and one or two personal points. Being a multi-faceted answer, you will need to keep each element succinct, as the tutor can always ask you to explain further. Below are some points outlined, that you could add to the above example.

"[University]'s faculty members, who have published some inspiring research (example), enable me to access studies from a unique angle, so far beyond simply reading the publication. I want to explore how the research process works for them, to enable me to better critique and publish my own research and writing, in a more comprehensive and well-rounded manner than I was able to in [e.g., EPQ]."

"As I discussed in my personal statement, I would love to pursue [insert career/academic goal]. Being surrounded by like-minded individuals and tutors who can push me to advance myself and my work will enable me to achieve that."

The second answer could have been *"Being surrounded by like-minded individuals will push me to achieve my goals."*. That would be a mediocre answer, whereas the example given provides colour to the generic point, making it personal to you. The key to this question is to not worry so much whether you answer is generic, but that it is true. Prove that truth by giving examples from your own personal life/studies/experiences.

Q19: Why do you want to study Experimental Psychology?

This is quite likely to be a warm-up question so you can use it to help the interviewer get to know you better. This answer is very similar to many of the 'why do you' questions, because the answer pool is mostly finite, meaning your ability to tune it to your own life is down to the personalisation. The first rule with this question is to know your subject. This includes course modules, exam structure, methods of assessment (dissertation, lab projects etc.) and a bit of subject knowledge. A key distinction to make in your mind is the difference between this question and *"Why is our experimental psychology course great?"*. It is totally fine to begin your answer by answering that questions, but the important bit is the 'you' bit. Here's an example of the former, without the latter.

"The course here covers [modules] which are really interesting, and the faculty building has an amazing library."

And here is the former, with the latter (the good bit) integrated in.

"The course here covers [modules], some of which I have begun studying during my A-Levels. A particular interest of mine is [module] which I have been focussing on recently, and this is something that isn't studied in a lot of (or any other, if you're lucky enough to find such a topic) psychology courses. The faculty building's library is large and always accessible; something I'm really keen to utilise, as I want to be able to study more effectively than I have been able to at home/school."

The core of the answer is the same, generic points, but the 'colour' given by the personalisation is what differentiates it from that generic answer. The best way to prepare this is to list some generic answers and see how you can apply them to yourself. If it's the truth, it'll come to mind much easier when you're asked about it than if it isn't!

Q20: Why do you want to come to this college?

Research is the key to this question. That doesn't mean just which faculty members are at the college, or how good the library is, think broader:

"How far is it from your department/favourite restaurant/tourist attraction?"

"Is it a quiet part of town?"

"Does it have nice grounds/views/areas to work outside?"

The risk with this question is that you stray too far into the titbits of information, without delving into the bigger points. Balancing these two is really important. If you spend your whole time talking about the library and faculty members, the answer will sound too over-rehearsed and devoid of personality. If you spend the whole time talking about the fact the college is over the road from your favourite restaurant, the answer will feel under-researched and without depth. Including both of these elements is key to a well-rounded answer. As with all 'why' questions, it is important to make sure you include as much personality and truth as you can. Here's an example of a well-research but poor answer.

"I would like to come to this college because it has the second biggest library of any college and the largest number of operating researchers in psychology. It's also the closest college to Mission Burrito, which is my favourite restaurant, and it's got the largest green space to total area ratio of all the colleges."

Here is an example using the same points, in a more personal and less rehearsed way.

"I would like to come to [college] for a few reasons. Firstly, are its facilities, I can see from the website that it has a huge library, so finding seats at busy times shouldn't be a problem. I've also read about the faculty members, lots of whom are psychology researchers; having the ability to meet with them more easily will be great for improving my research and writing skills. I've also looked on a map of Oxford and seen that it has big green spaces, which will be great for relaxing in during downtime when the weather is nice. Lastly, it's really close to my favourite restaurant, Mission Burrito, which will make the longer working days a bit easier!"

The second answer still follows the list-like format of the first, making it easier to keep track of when talking (helping you not to drift off-topic), without sounding like you're reading it off of the college Wikipedia page! Each point references a reason for liking the college, so you're combining the answers to *"Why is this college good?"* and *"Why do you like this college?"*.

Q21: Describe phantom limb syndrome?

With a scientific question like this, which addresses a specific condition, it is important to address that first. If you don't know the condition, that's fine. The important thing is that you make the interviewer aware of that immediately with your answer. The worst thing you can do is spend a minute wandering your thoughts around the answer. Below is an example of not addressing the question, which might be quite tempting if you do not know the answer and wish to disguise that.

"There are lots of medical conditions that can affect the limbs. Some of them can make the sufferer unstable on their feet, or struggle to do basic tasks like dress themselves. There are some conditions which might be invisible and some which are very obvious, the former are often more harmful to the sufferer's mental health. I am sure phantom limb syndrome can negatively affect all kinds of people."

If you were to answer like this, the interviewer will see, in a few moments, that you don't know the answer. Or, they might think you don't know how to concisely answer a scientific question. However, if you address your lack of knowledge immediately, you can create a much more mature and impactful answer, such as that below.

"I don't know exactly what phantom limb syndrome is. However, I can guess that it affects the limbs, or perhaps the sufferer's perception of their limbs. The word phantom suggests that the condition might not be physical, so it could be a condition with symptoms similar to that which some sufferers of anorexia have, whereby their vision of their body is distorted from reality. Perhaps someone with phantom limb syndrome sees their limbs differently to how they appear in reality, maybe bigger or perhaps with a skin condition."

You can see, if you were to google phantom limb syndrome (or know what it was already), that the answer here is completely wrong. However, that doesn't matter as much as how you present your answer. You can see that the respondent's knowledge of the syndrome is immediately addressed by explaining they do not know exactly what the syndrome is. They then think aloud, using the information they have to deduce an answer that makes sense to them. This is a similar process to which you might undertake when understanding something in a lecture, tutorial or a research paper. Sometimes, looking something up is impractical/unprofessional, or perhaps you simply do not have the means by which to do so at that moment. In those instances, it is important to have the ability to make an educated guess, which you can confirm later on.

Remember, if you do know the answer, make sure you provide and concise explanation. Don't be afraid to ask the tutor questions, if there are elements to your answer that you are not certain of, or believe can be expanded upon. That insight is more important than your knowledge of the specific topic.

Q22: How would you approach treating phantom limb syndrome?

This is a question which requires very specific scientific knowledge to answer correctly, not something that would typically be expected of you in an interview scenario. The first thing to do in this situation is assess whether or not you are confident in knowing the answer. If you are, go ahead and provide a concise explanation. Don't be afraid to ask the tutor questions, if there are elements to your answer that you are not certain of or believe can be expanded upon. That insight is more important than your knowledge of the specific topic.

If you are not sure of the answer to a question like this, ask questions first. The point of this question is to answer how you treat this syndrome so, if you don't know what the syndrome is, ask that first. The interviewer may be happy to tell you, and you can build your answer from there. If they are not willing to answer any questions, make sure you think aloud. An example of this is the answer below.

"I am not sure what phantom limb syndrome is, however, it is clear that it affects the limbs. Or, perhaps the sufferer's perception of their limbs. The word phantom suggests that the syndrome might not be real or manifest physically. One option is perhaps that the syndrome results in a sufferer who has lost a limb, thinking that it is still there, perhaps by means of hallucinations. One way to treat this could be by taking them through the timeline that led to the loss of their limb, or perhaps showing them photos or video where you can see them without the limb. If someone is hallucinating, the broader cause of the condition may be entirely different, and the phantom limb syndrome is just a biproduct of something larger. Treating a broader condition like that might require drug intervention."

If you were to look up phantom limb syndrome (or know what it is already), you'd know that the answer above is not quite right. However, the answer immediately addresses the lack of knowledge and then proceeds to demonstrate the respondents thought process by thinking aloud through their logical steps. It is always okay to ask questions, but don't be put off if the interviewer tells you they can't answer them. This isn't indicative of you not knowing something that you should, it is simply the interviewer guiding you towards the thought process they want to observe you undertaking.

Q23: What made you choose psychology over a related subject like medicine?

Answering this question can be approached in two ways, depending on whether or not you considered medicine as an option. If you did consider medicine as an option, then you can stick primarily to honest answers about your decision process. It would be best to avoid answers like *"medicine had higher entry requirements"* or *"I didn't study the right A-Levels for medicine"* because these give off a sense of unpreparedness and lack of consideration during your previous studies. Better answers are ones that consider the future and demonstrate that you have given thought to the decisions you have made so far. Here is an example of one possible, good answer.

"I didn't apply for medicine because my interest in psychology has already led me to pursue a career in the field. Studying psychology rather than medicine will allow me to specialise earlier on and pursue a more specific field of psychology in post-graduate studies, having a greater depth of specific knowledge to base that from."

That answer demonstrates that the respondent is confident in their decision to study psychology, has a plan for the future, and has considered why psychology is a better option for them than medicine. While this answer would be satisfactory, it would be better to have some more extensive knowledge of subjects alongside (but which may be related to) psychology. It is possible that an interviewer may ask a question like this to pry into your depth of knowledge around the course content. Here, they are looking for your understanding of what the degree course focusses on, and perhaps things that it misses out. For example, at Oxford you can study Experimental Psychology or Psychology, Philosophy and Linguistics. For an Oxford application, it would be important to understand the difference between these subjects and their course content. In an ideal world, you would pick out one or two modules which are unique to the course that you have chosen and discuss why they are of particular interest to you. The more closely you can relate this to future plans or past experiences (like in the above example), the better. Whichever specific subject or university you are applying for, have a look to see if your chosen subject has any 'sister-subjects' and try to find some differences to highlight.

Q24: Here's a graph showing the perception of pain against stimulation - why does perception of pain level off while stimulation continues to increase at the top?

At first glance this question seems like it requires biology/neurophysiology knowledge, something that you may have from reading around the subject of psychology. However, while that knowledge certainly will help, you don't need it to answer this question well. The first thing to remember, as with almost every interview question, is to make sure you verbalise your thought processes. Start at the highest possible level you can consider; in this case, what is pain for? Pain is there to warn you against doing something again, or to indicate to you that something is wrong. If you do something that breaks your skin, you risk infection or blood-loss, so nerves give you a pain signal which tells you that whatever action has led to this is not something you should repeat. Here's an example of how you might start at that high-level and explore the question.

"Pain exists to warn you against doing something, or to indicate that something is wrong. Therefore, its purpose lies in the acute response, rather than the chronic. As a result, it would make sense for pain to become severe quickly, to act as a warning, but stop at a certain point to avoid incapacitating you. If you are incapacitated by pain, you are unable to physically act to avoid the cause of the pain, this is counter-intuitive in many cases."

You might then choose to explore the biological aspect of this.

"Nerves communicate by sending signals across synapses very quickly, so this pattern could be achieved by the initial receiving of these signals generating the rapidly rising pain response. However, if these signals continue to be received, it makes little sense to keep raising the pain response beyond a certain point, so maybe the areas of the nerve that receive the signal become saturated."

This answer has required very little knowledge of nerves, essentially only that a synapse (although you need not know the technical term) is the bridge between neurons and they can send/receive physical 'signals'. However, by exploring both elements you have demonstrating your knowledge of psychology, your application of psychology to a biological setting, and your deductive thinking when making that connection. The answer ends up being well-rounded and comprehensive, as well as demonstrating your competent thought processes, without requiring anything more than very basic pre-reading knowledge and no specialist vocabulary.

Q25: How would you model the brain?

The first thing to address with this question is the purpose of the model. You can ask the question or, if you like, address that a model can be for many purposes and consider a few individually. Some ideas include; a representation of the external physiology of the brain, a model which can be taken apart to show the internal construction of the brain or a reductionist model that represents simply the brain's size/texture/weight.

It is probably best to then begin your explanation with a very brief address of the reductionist model, perhaps a material suggestion (e.g., silicon) and a method (if you can think of one) you could use to actually construct it. You don't want to spend long on these simplistic explanations as it will appear that you don't have material to delve into the more complex and important elements. When addressing the ideal of a physiologically representative model of the brain, you want to express your knowledge of the brain's construction and relate that to the difficulties in physically creating that. A suggestion is below.

"The brain is made up of grey and white matter, which is constructed from many millions of interconnected neurons. Building a model of this would require very finely tuned tools, certainly a computer-based system to construct it. If you wished to construct a physiologically accurate representation, you would have to scan one person's brain and base it on that, as every brain is different."

At this point, you could go on and discuss ways in which you could scan the brain, however, you will not necessarily be expected to have explicit knowledge of the different types of brains scans (although, as with all of this extra knowledge, it can't hurt!). In the case that you do not know any specific scan types, or which one would be appropriate, then go on to explain what you would need from the scan.

"The scan would need to be 3-dimensional and have a very high resolution to capture the neuronal layout. However, the resolution would need only be as high as the machine that will build the model, unless then scan is going to be used for something else too. Some scans might take into account movement of signals, this one would not as the model will be static."

The most important thing with a question like this is that you understand the limitations of what you are doing and make suggestions of how to overcome them (if appropriate). When it comes to something like scan resolution, which cannot be changed, then simply acknowledge the consequence of that. In this case, the model will not likely be truly representative of a brain as it cannot contain every neuron individually. Remember, a model can be digital so you could always add that if it were not required to be physical, then you could take multiple scans and stitch them together in a digital model, to increase the resolution and accuracy.

Q26: Why are faces so important?

There are a dozen ways in which you could approach this question. However, you need to consider it from a psychological standpoint, as that is what the interviewer will be interested in. When considering something 'from a psychological standpoint', always consider perception. We see faces as a way of recognising someone and that is based on their uniqueness. However, someone's hand is also usually in view when with somebody and is just as unique as their face, yet you wouldn't likely be able to recognise an old friend by their hand. When starting to answer a question like this, always articulate your thought process aloud. This enables the interviewer to see the unique way in which you have come to your discussion point, but also to guide you in a different direction if they feel you are straying from the point of the question. At the end of the day, the interviewer wants to have a good discussion with you. Otherwise, you wouldn't have been invited for interview!

Once you have outlined your thought process, you should then approach explicitly answering the question. While it sounds obvious, it is a common mistake to talk around the subject rather than explicitly answering the question, in the same way as you might when writing an essay! When discussing what makes a face special, you must address both what is special about it (in your current line of discussion) and what is it that makes that aspect special in the first place. Following on from the line of thought in the first paragraph, the thing that is special about a face is its recognisability. The next part of the discussion is how that comes about.

"One thing that makes a face special is others' ability to recognise someone by it, in spite of the fact it is no more unique than many other parts of the body, like hands. One explanation for this could be that the features of a face are more obvious because they are very three-dimensional, on the front of the head, and at eye level. This makes differences easier to notice than differences on a hand."

That is one reason why a face is special, with one explanation for how that speciality could have come to be. There are many ways in which a face is special, but you can apply this formula of explanation to any of your ideas. There are no wrong answers here, providing they are thought-out and justified. This type of question is a test of thinking on your feet, you are very unlikely to have any form of prepared answer due to the vast number of different topics the interviewer could choose from!

Q27: What did you find interesting about the book you read?

When answering this question, the interviewer is testing two things. Firstly, that you have actually read what you say you have read (whether that be from your personal statement or from name-dropping a book in a previous conversation). The interviewer may not know anything about the book (which means you could make up pretty much what you want!), or they may know it word for word. I'd bet on the latter so be prepared!

The first step to answering this question is to actually explain the section of the book you wish to talk about. It might be an experiment, a character/biographical section, an event, or something else entirely. The important thing is that you find it interesting and you know it well enough to explain it! It would be best to have read a book that has a psychology aspect to it, as this will be easiest to engage the tutor with. However, that is not a requirement (unless it is specifically a book you were asked to read to gain subject knowledge) and you are welcome to talk about something less related. It is, however, difficult to bring the message of an unrelated topic into the context of a psychology interview. By picking something psychology-related, you do also demonstrate that your interest is piqued by subject-matter, which is definitely a good thing in the eyes of a tutor!

When discussing an interesting point, you want to explain the point first, before outlining why it is interesting. This order makes the initial explanation more engaging, and helps you avoid repeating yourself, wandering off-topic or losing your train of thought. What you want to avoid, is simply explaining why you find the topic interesting from a non-specific or an overly personal way (anecdotes are fine, but try to keep them psychology related in some way). An example of a poor explanation for why something is interesting is below.

"I found that study interesting because I'm a real cat lover, and getting to explore the mind of a cat in that way really engaged me"

A better way to express that, while maintaining the personal touch, could be as follows.

"I found that study interesting because it explored the mind of a cat. Lots of other studies I have read have looked at feline brain chemistry or physiology, but not the actual cognitive processes. As a cat lover, it's also fun to get to peek into their minds!"

By opening with the scientific aspect, and keeping the anecdote related, you can construct a more mature and convincing answer. Make sure you focus on one point in this question, the interviewer is not trying to test your recall of the entire book, just your interest in one part.

Q28: What is the appeal of experimental psychology to you personally?

As with all questions that address the subject you are applying for directly, there is an underlying assessment happening of your course knowledge. When answering this question, try to keep that in mind for at least some of your points. There may be some exclusively personal points you want to make, which is fine, as long as they are supplemented with ones that demonstrate you have read up on the course content. Unless you have particular reason to open with a point unrelated to the course content, it might be wise to begin with that. It will likely relax the interviewer somewhat as they can see you are well-read and will likely be less focussed on assessing that from future points you make.

When considering a point with a course content focus, it would be best to avoid simply listing some modules and stating that you are excited to learn them. This demonstrates a very limited appreciation of the course content, and scream 'last minute cram' before you walked in. You're far better off picking one or two modules and explaining why they appeal to you in more detail. Try to pick modules that might be less likely to occur in other psychology courses; think 'experimental'. One example could be as follows.

"The core practical element of the course is something that greatly appeals to me. I am excited not only to explore and undertake experiments of my own, but also to get access to the tools and techniques that researchers use to design and perform studies. I am excited by the prospect of coding my own statistical analyses, as I am really enjoying the manual statistics I'm currently completing in A-Level maths. The opportunity to utilise tools like MATLAB to explore those analyses in a more complicated way and with larger datasets is really appealing."

Your answer will almost certainly be better by outlining more than one element of the course that interests you, as well as a personal aspect. However, it is far better to go into the detail like the above answer on one point, than it is to simply list off many modules or make a few comparisons to the A-Level course.

Q29: Take a look at this data from a psychology experiment - how would you try to interpret this?

Answering a question like this is all down to your thinking process. As ever, it is vital that you make this process an aloud one, so the interviewer can follow along and appreciate the steps you are taking. If you give a 'wrong' answer, you want the interviewer to understand why, and appreciate how the thought process went awry, rather than simply hearing a wrong answer without context. When given data, you want to point out absolutely everything you notice, starting with the simplest. Firstly, this demonstrates to the interviewer that you are considering all variables and points of observation. Just as importantly however, the sooner you get your brain on the task, the sooner you'll be fully engaged. If you don't understand what is put in front of you, it's very easy to just stare blankly at it as you try to understand the bigger picture from moment one.

If the data is in the form of a graph, there are lots of different aspects of the graph to address. When addressing them, try to contextualise any of the points where there might be a motivation behind what has been done. For example, some graphs don't start at zero on one or either of their axes. This is something great to point out, but an even better answer will be one that considers why this is.

"The y axis on this graph starts at 6 rather than 0. This could be to make the difference between variable A and B appear larger, because you cannot see the full height of the graph."

This is a great answer, but an excellent answer would be to expand on this by contextualising it in the real world of using data.

"One reason for doing this might be to make the point the presenter wants to make, appear to be more supported by the graph than it is. This could be to exaggerate the effectiveness of an intervention, in order to present it as successful."

By exploring the data to this depth, you are demonstrating your observation/understanding of data and the ways in which it is presented, what the consequences of different presentation types are, and human motivations behind these actions.

Q30: Do you think computers could ever be as complicated as a human brain?

As with many scientific questions, there are terms within them which need clarification before proceeding. It is up to your discretion whether you choose one definition and go with it, or address the fact there are multiple definitions and address some/all of them. In this case, the world 'complex' is ambiguous. Complexity in this context could refer to the number of neurons in the brain, how each of those neurons function, the degree to which the neurons are interconnected, the underlying cell structure of the brain as a whole, or even the complexity of the outputs which can be produced by the human brain.

To address all of these would be more of an essay than an answer to an interview question. If you believe you could address them all in a concise manner, then you would be welcome to do so, the interviewer may even encourage you to do so after you have outlined them. If you have outlined a large number of points such as this, and you have somewhere to write them down, it might be a good idea to do so. It would be a shame to lose out on an interesting discussion because you have forgotten the starting point!

Alternatively, you could only discuss one or two of these points. Whether you do this, or address all of them, it is a good idea to outline as many as you can think of in the beginning. This demonstrates comprehensive understanding and thinking which exhausts all options; both traits which an interviewer will want to see in you. In theory, every point of consideration should generate a slightly different answer.

"If complexity is defined as the number of individual sections, then yes, we probably can make a computer as complex as the human brain. We can fit billions of transistors on to a tiny microchip, so if we had a computing unit the size of a human brain, we could almost certainly have as many transistors as the brain does neurons, or even cells. However, if complexity is measured by the number of outputs, then the answer is less clear. Theoretically, the human brain can output an infinite number of responses – hence why every person is unique. However, that theory can also stretch to a computer's outputs. With that in mind, it depends on whether you consider infinite to be a valid measure."

While the actual train of discussion may continue on longer than that above, this demonstrates a way in which you can concisely address two of the outlined points. These two were picked because they don't directly align. It would be best not to discuss two points which have the same conclusion, as it would make it much harder to avoid repeating yourself!

Q31: What is the most interesting thing about Psychology?

This question is a chance to both be honest, but also to demonstrate your subject and course knowledge. An ideal answer will outline some elements of the psychological discipline which genuinely interest you, which you will study in the course to which you are applying, and which will lead you to a plan for the future/study focus in your later degree years. Finding an answer such as this is incredibly difficult and not everyone will have one, but you want to try and satisfy as many of these as possible, with the order they are written here being their order of importance.

Firstly, you should be discussing an element that interests you. To discuss this with conviction, you should have some kind of reason for that interest. As long as it is honest, it doesn't need to be elaborate, but the more weight it can carry the better. A good example of this would be as follows.

"I am particularly interested in the science of addiction. I find it fascinating that it's a clear demonstration of the interaction between behaviour and brain chemistry and is something we can observe to a degree in almost everyone."

A bad example is below.

"I am particularly interested in the science of addiction. I find it fascinating because of how common it is in people."

Without the foundation in scientific theory, the answer sounds entirely unprepared and lacking conviction.

Picking an element, and presenting it in this way, that is a part of the course (e.g., a module) is a great way of implying your course knowledge again, reinforcing this message to the tutor without having to explicitly recite course content. Lastly, if you have a particular interest in a topic and would want to write a dissertation on it, study it experimentally, or even work in the field after university, say so! Not everyone has things planned that far ahead, and the tutors won't expect you to. However, if you have, they'll be very impressed that you've tied all this together!

Q32: Does phenotype depend on nature or nurture?

The nature-nurture argument is fundamental in psychology and will be the backbone of many discussions through your degree. The first thing to consider is whether you know what a phenotype is, as it may not be a word you have come across/remember if you have not studied psychology or biology at A-Level. It's ok to ask the interviewer a question like this, as it is fundamental to your ability to create an answer. However, you should make sure that you have suitably read-up by the time the interview comes around, such that you know terms like this. A great way to 'read-up' on the basics is to go through the glossary of a psychology textbook and read the definitions of any words you do not know. You will never remember all of them, but it will help you get familiar with the vocabulary.

Once you know what phenotype means, you have then got to construct an answer which considers both sides. Just like in an essay, you want to spend some time addressing both nature and nurture, with the focus being on the one you believe to be true (or simply, more true/likely). Once you have discussed both sides, make sure to conclude. It is very easy to tail off at the end of a discussion, so make sure you round off with a clear conclusion (even if you have not made a decision, make that indecision the conclusion!). The easiest way to make sure you follow this structure, is to clearly segment your argument from the beginning. This is an example of a basic, but clear, way to start an answer.

"As with many nature nurture arguments, there are valid views on both sides. One way in which phenotypes could be considered nature is that their expression is decided, in origin, by the genotype we possess. This is something built into our DNA and is pre-decided before we are born."

While it might seem too reductionist to begin an answer with such a cut and dry way of speaking, it is a great way to simply let the tutor know that you are going to be considering both sides, and that you are starting with one. You can then go on to make a few points for this argument, a few for the other (making it clear when you change), and then conclude. The most important thing about the conclusion is you include one! Don't worry if it doesn't actually make any kind of strong decision!

Q33: Do you think you are born with a high IQ, or develop one?

While it does not explicitly state it, this question is a nature-nurture argument question. As with any of these questions, it is important to discuss both sides and then make a clear conclusion. The conclusion doesn't have to decide anything, indecision in itself is just as valid a conclusion! An understanding of exactly what IQ measures, and how it is calculated/compared would be useful to answer this question. However, if you don't know either of those things, you have two options. You can either proceed with the assumption that IQ simply measures general intelligence and not consider how it is compared between people, or you could choose to ask the interviewer to explain the concept in some more detail. With a question like this, where the term is ubiquitously known and not strictly psychology-related, it might be more fluid to start with an initial discussion and then ask if you get stuck/run out of ideas.

When considering whether someone is born with their IQ, it is important to make this more comprehensive a point, by outlining how that would have come about. If IQ is entirely nature-decided, then your genetic makeup is what decides your IQ and this is inherited by your parents. This would suggest that only people with high-IQ parents would have high IQ's. However, always consider further when making blanket statements like this. What if combining two high-IQ genotypes, creates a genotype that decides you have a low IQ? What about mistakes in RNA copying? There are many questions you can explore, depending on how in-depth your biological knowledge is regarding genetics. It is important to remember that you do not need to know the answer to ask the question, it is always better to simply demonstrate that you are considering the point.

When considering IQ as a nurture-decided feature of a person, have a think about all the factors that come into it. This is everything from the potentially obvious e.g., education, to the further afield e.g., dietary quality/variety as a child. As with so many of these questions, the most important thing is to consider as many factors as possible, regardless of whether you know the answer at the end. Practicing answering questions like this will help you learn to organise these thoughts and present them in a coherent way.

Q34: What is sentience? Prove to me that you are sentient.

With any two-part question, it is vital that you split up the two parts. This doesn't necessarily mean giving two fully separated answers (although this is sometimes the best way to do it), but you must make two distinct conclusions at the very least. The first question is an abstract philosophy question, while the second one can be more closely attuned to a psychology answer.

When answering a question like this first one, it is very easy to drift away from the point and have a general discussion around the topic. Therefore, to avoid this, you should try to make your initial definition concise (you can always consider an alternative definition later on!). It is important to keep your psychology 'head' on when answering this sort of question. The more references you can make to psychology material when answering, the better!

"Sentience could be considered from a philosophical, psychological or biological standpoint. Is consciousness an awareness of oneself, or perhaps a recognition of others also having thoughts? Or could sentience be a particular arrangement of neurons that make decisions?"

By addressing the different options for consideration at the beginning, you are pre-structuring your argument. This makes it much easier to return to 'home' in your thought process and embark on exploring another point from there. This creates an argument that is both easier to follow, and which likely covers the material more comprehensively. Having these different points also makes it easier to transition into answering the second question. For example, if considering this from the philosophical standpoint, perhaps the very fact you can consider your own sentience is enough to confirm that you are conscious. However, from a biological standpoint, you cannot possibly be aware of your physical brain make-up unless you have a brain scan, and it would be entirely illogical to consider that being the point at which you become sentient. Exploring the topic in this deconstructed way enables you to be comprehensive in your discussion and sets you up for making the all-important conclusion!

Q35: Can fish hear sound?

This question, despite its simplicity is testing three things, all of different importance. The first is your understanding of fish physiology and behaviour (the least important), secondly is your understanding of what sound is, and lastly is your understanding of how these compare to human physiology (because we definitely do hear sound!)

If you know anything about fish physiology, then feel free to open with it! These sorts of titbits of information can bring some personality to the interview experience and make the interviewer remember you! However, the real test comes in the second part, which is your understanding of sound. The interviewer will expect you to know the very basic fact that sound is a wave (GCSE physics!), and the fact that soundwaves can travel underwater (whale songs!). Anything beyond this is a bonus, the important bit is how you compare this to the human experience. However, it is vital to remember that the question's conclusion needs to be answering the question, not comparing fish to humans!

"Humans hear sound by using tiny bones in our ears to receive sound waves. These waves are interpreted as sound and transformed using neural signals, into something we 'hear'. Fish could have this biological setup, and sound travels underwater in a similar way, so from this standpoint fish could definitely hear sound."

This answer fully explains your understanding of the physiology around how we hear and compares it to your knowledge of fish. But, most importantly, it concludes by answering the actual question, rather than concluding on the human comparison! Depending on your knowledge of a topic like this, your answer could vary in length greatly. Feel free to explore some things you are not sure of, but make sure you keep the answer to a reasonably concise length and have a conclusion at the end. The interviewer can always (and probably will) ask more questions if they want to continue the discussion!

Q36: What marks the boundary between neuroscience and psychology?

This is a very important question to clearly distinguish between the terms, and how the concepts are treated in the real world. In the reality of studying either of these subjects, there will be overlap. However, that does not mean that the terms overlap. It would be incorrect to make a sweeping statement, such as 'neuroscience is physical, and psychology is abstract/conceptual' unless you are sure that your definition is correct. This is a closed answer and invites the interviewer to directly disagree with you (which, even if they don't view it as a bad thing, might throw you off!). To answer a question which's foci are both actual terms and concepts/subjects, it is important to explain the distinction.

"When studying psychology, neurophysiology serves to supplement many of the studies and theories. One example of this is, when considering the interpretation of brain signals, you must know in what form those signals manifest and how they are transported! However, when it comes to defining them, there may be a clearer distinction. For example, you might consider something to transition from psychology to neurophysiology (written this way to reflect the 'psychology ending and neurophysiology beginning' phrasing of the question) *when it becomes physically represented."*

You can see from the example answer, that the conclusion of psychology and neurophysiology being differentiated by their physical/non-physical nature is the same as the sweeping statement from the first paragraph. However, by using a precursory discussion and a less definitive statement, the answer invites discussion rather than a disagreement.

If you want to explore the question more deeply, it can be helpful to ask the interviewer to repeat the question after your first discussion point. After hearing the question again, you may pick up on the 'psychology ending and neurophysiology beginning' element. One way to consider this, is to explore how you would study something in these two subjects. With a concept like pain, you could approach it from two angles. The first would be to measure signals in the brain and assess how they are manifested as physical and non-physical reactions, such as feelings (the psychological part). The alternative, is to consider pain from a psychological standpoint (e.g., loss) and consider how that manifests in a physical form. By comparing the physical pain and its associated signals, along with emotional pain and its associated signals, you can begin to differentiate between the two concepts. Considering that psychology 'ends' when neurophysiology 'begins', suggests that the concepts may be differentiated by their approach angle. Psychology could be considered the study of non-physical manifestations of brain signals, while neurophysiology is the physical manifestation of brain signals. The interesting point to consider becomes whether you see brain signals as the electrical pulses they are, or the reactions generated by your brain to create behaviour/emotion etc.

Q37: What effect does heroin have on the brain?

As is the case with scientific questions such as this, the more you know the better. However, lots of prior knowledge is not necessary to answer it well. An interviewer will not expect you to have lots of prior knowledge on a particular subject, unless it is part of your pre-reading, or you have mentioned it in your personal statement/other interviews. If you don't have specific knowledge, then there has to be a process of deduction.

If you know that heroin is addictive, and you know that someone who takes heroin would have withdrawal symptoms if they stopped taking it, that's a great start to assessing what it does to the brain. One way in which something can become addictive, is by making you feel good when you use it. Opioids are one chemical that can make you feel good and happen to be heroin's source of the 'feel good' response. You don't need to know the chemical name, but some extra vocabulary is always helpful to make the answer you give clearer. The important part of this question is how you use the little knowledge you have to create a more comprehensive answer.

"Heroin gives a 'feel-good' feeling by flooding the brain with opioid chemicals. This would activate all the neurons with opioid receptors and generate a feeling of euphoria. However, as with pain receptors only receiving the pain signals up to a certain point, there must be a limit to how many receivers there are, and therefore be a point at which they become entirely saturated. At that point, there is no longer any reason for the body to generate its own opioids, so it stops. As a result, once the effects of the heroin wear off, there are no opioids to replace the synthetic ones. As a result, you could become depressed and crave the good feeling that taking heroin brought. In addition, because your 'default state' is now no opioids, rather than just a normal amount, the feeling that heroin brings becomes a more extreme version of happiness than it was originally, making you crave that feeling even more."

As you can see in this answer, the scientific knowledge required is very minimal, and the exact science behind the suggested is not even exactly correct. The point is that you have taken some very minor scientific insight and applied it to a situation, to explain an effect that you know exists. In the real world, you could look up any of the specific knowledge, so the interviewer is really testing your deductive thinking and your ability to apply knowledge. Remember though, if the topic is mentioned in your personal statement, or in some reading you have discussed, expect the interviewer to want more than the most basic knowledge from you!

Q38: Do you agree with Freud?

Freud being as famous as he is in the psychology community, you would be expected to have at least some very basic insight into his theories. Two over-arching theories of his are the concept of the unconscious mind (a space of thoughts in the brain that the conscious mind is not immediately aware of) and the idea of the three-part personality, made up of the Id, Ego and Superego. Freud had many more theories, lots of which with their own controversies. You would be welcome to discuss as many as you know, however these two are some broad and fundamental principles.

The unconscious mind is linked to events such as a 'Freudian slip', when you accidentally say something aloud that you did not mean to. This could be calling someone by the wrong name, or 'speaking before you think'. Freud believed that these events occurred because the unconscious mind was feeding into your expression. It's important, in cases such as these, that you distinguish between the reality of the event, and the proposed reason for it. Everyone has said something they didn't mean to at some point, and it would be very easy to believe that the source of that thought was the unconscious mind. However, just because a theory makes sense with the evidence you have, does not mean it's correct. This is a fundamental principle in scientific theory-making. You can never prove something in science, it is only as-yet uncontested. The more evidence you can gather in its favour, and the more you can dismiss that goes against it, the more confident you can be in that theory's reliability.

"Everyone has said something they didn't mean to and weren't aware they were about to. While these are the typical characteristics of a 'Freudian slip', it does not mean that Freud's theory is necessarily correct. The origin of these thoughts could have been from a memory or thought that was simply not being accessed in that moment, because you were concentrating on speaking. There is not necessarily this entirely separate and inaccessible part of the mind that Freud proposed to exist."

This answer addresses an important part of Freud's theory, acknowledges how it might have come about, but discusses an alternative interpretation of the phenomenon in question. It is important to know that Freud is largely discredited in the psychology world, so the interviewer will be quite surprised if you go ahead and agree with Freud explicitly. If you have the evidence, and the coherence of argument to agree, then you would be welcome to. These concepts are exactly that, concepts, and there is no 'proof' as to which theory is correct. There are, of course, more modern studies that provide different theories and interpretations of events, but that isn't to mean that some of the older theories don't have truth to them. The important thing is that you consider any evidence you have to hand, and make sure you provide some kind of alternative suggestion if you are going to disagree.

Q39: Can machines think?

Artificial intelligence is very likely to be a topic approached by your interviewers at some point. The concepts around it are very new in the world of psychology, so there are many unanswered questions. When answering a conceptual question which hinges on an action of some kind, in this case that action is making a decision, it is vital that you define that action. When it comes to making a decision, the important concept is not that it can decide between two options, but exactly where a 'decision' originates.

Making a decision could be considered from a very pragmatic point of view, being that you are given a number of options to weigh up, and you act in the direction of one of them. If that is where your definition of decision ends, then it would be logical to assume that machines can make decisions. For example, your phone 'chooses' to turn off when it gets too hot. It has the option to turn off or to continue working and it 'decides' to switch off. The difference is an understanding of why that decision is being made. When explaining this to someone, you might say that your phone turns itself off to protect it from overheating (and potentially damaging its components). However, that isn't why it does it at all. The person who programmed it, programmed it to do that for that reason. However, the phone turns off because a particular thermometer (or other related measuring device) reaches a certain temperature (or other temperature-related signal). The act of turning off has nothing to do with self-protection because the phone has no concept of that.

"Having discussed how acting one particular way in a situation is different to the typical way in which we might consider a human (or animal) makes a decision, the question becomes how you define decision. If you consider a decision to be an action based on a measured response to a situation, the machines definitely can make decisions and do not need to be 'intelligent' to do so. However, if a decision relies on the ability for the decision-maker to understand the reason for and the consequence of their decision, beyond simply the measured variables, then that becomes a much more difficult question."

In this answer, you have ensured that the question has been answered explicitly (in this case, according to one definition of decision), but also made sure the interviewer is aware that you have considered the concept to a deeper level. The latter is important, as it will likely provoke further interviewer engagement and conversation, which is a great sign that they are interested in what you are saying! You do not necessarily need to answer the additional concept that you propose, unless explicitly asked to, but make sure that you outline it. If you do go down the route of attempting to answer it, just make sure you stay on-topic and don't drift too far afield from the question.

Q40: Would you give chimpanzees human rights?

When discussing the concept of 'rights' the important point to address is why those rights have been given to whoever (or whatever) has them. In the case of humans and chimpanzees, there are some distinct differences and similarities to be addressed. On the one hand, chimpanzees are categorically not humans and, therefore, should have no reason to be treated as such. With that in mind, there may be many rights that a chimpanzee should have for other reasons, but they should not be 'human' rights. On the other hand, chimpanzees are emotionally intelligent, forward-thinking and can 'feel', so they should have human rights. The important distinction to make is whether human rights are referred to as such simply because they are rights for humans, or whether they are human concepts.

For some rights, it appears quite clear. One human right is the right to education, something that it would seem obvious to be not applicable to chimpanzees. However, this would only be if we consider education to be a formal human education. Chimpanzees are all 'educated' by their parents, on how to hunt/forage/defend themselves etc. it would make no sense to enforce human education on to chimpanzees, but it would make sense to ensure all chimpanzees live in groups, so that they can educate each other in this way. An extension to this concept would be to allow chimpanzees to live in a 'wild setting', in order that they can continue to learn these ways of living and pass it on to their own offspring.

As you can see, even a right which appears to be clearly linked to humans is not clear when you delve into the concepts behind it. It becomes even more complicated when you consider the definition of education from a human standpoint. A human rights activist wouldn't likely consider a human to having their human right to education met, if they were raised in a 'wild setting' and simply taught how to forage and defend themselves. Therefore, it is clear that the definition of each concept is very important. This brings the argument full-circle back to whether human rights are as such because they are rights that apply to humans, or whether it is because they are human concepts.

As suggested here, it is very easy to become lost in one aspect of this question. The important thing to remember is that you should always address the question directly at the end of each discussion element. If you choose to discuss human rights by one definition, answer the question based on that definition before moving on to an alternative. Not only does this bring some structure and clarity to your answer, but it gives the interviewer an opportunity to step in and guide the discussion in a particular direction of their interest.

CHEMISTRY

In your interviews, your knowledge of a range of topics could be tested as well as your ability to apply your understanding of specific cases to other situations. The questions could be drawn from any part of the curriculum, so there is no way to revise just the area you will be tested on. There is no specific way to prepare for the example types of questions given in this chapter, or the similar styles of question that could be derived from other parts of the curriculum. The important thing is to have a **sound understanding of not just specific instances you have rote-learned for exams, but the chemical principles that underlie them**. When you do your revision for your interview, make sure you always ask why certain results are achieved – don't just learn that a certain compound is less reactive, make sure you know why that is. If you don't know, then ask your teacher about the underlying principles, or even better, try to figure out the answer yourself to practice this way of thinking.

For instance, you could be asked questions about chemical formulae and their relation to structure and physical or chemical properties. For this style of question, you may be asked to **draw the chemical formula** for an ionic compound and a covalent compound, and then asked to draw the formula for something in-between like Al_3O_6. You could also be asked to draw in detail each atom with electrons and describe their distribution in the shells and Bohr's theories explaining this behaviour.

Alternatively, you could be asked to draw an organic compound from the formula and asked about the physical properties you would expect. This could be a compound you are expected to be familiar with. Then, you could be asked to draw other compounds with similar properties, or how you would alter the original compound for a new property. You could be given a made up chemical formula and be asked to draw a suggestion for how it may be structured to have certain properties. You could be questioned about the **nature of any bonds** or how properties might change for enantiomers.

Your knowledge around the subject might be tested by asking about a well-known case, such as Thalidomide or hydrocarbon fractionation. Moving away from chemical structures and properties, you could be asked **calculation-based questions** such as molar equations or thermodynamics (entropy and enthalpy, reaction rates, phase changes, etc.). Given the nature of the interview, you are unlikely to get an in-depth calculation-based question.

However, knowledge of these topics might be necessary to answer questions such as: How would you balance these reactions? Which reaction would proceed faster? Which reaction would you expect to occur spontaneously? Would you expect either to reach equilibrium? Which conditions would you alter to change your answer? The important thing is not to have the right answer, but to show you can reason through unfamiliar examples using your knowledge of the principles.

As it is an experimental subject, your knowledge of experimental techniques and examples could be tested. Make sure you **revise the material and methods used in experiments and practicals**, in case you are asked specific questions about designing an experiment or interpreting results. An example of this is being asked to design an experiment to identify an unknown organic acid. This might involve an understanding of titration curves for mono-, di-, and tri-protic acids and how to generate them in the lab, or a number of other topics you may have covered in experiments.

As an extension of this, be familiar with the techniques that were used to discover the facts and theories in your textbooks as you could be asked how they were discovered or how you would verify they are true.

WORKED QUESTIONS

Below are a few examples of how to start breaking down an interview question, complete with model answers. They are by no means an exhaustive list but they give a sense of how A-level material can be used as a basis for questions that require independent thought and problem-solving skills. Use these examples as a guide of what topics to revise and the style of questions that may arise.

Q1: How did we find out the composition of the sun?

This is a common example, so you may be expected to be somewhat familiar with it. Don't be discouraged if you are not though, the interviewer may be even more impressed if you can reach a reasonable answer all on your own. The gist of this question is to use spectral analysis and knowledge of the theories underlying it to determine the sun's composition using its own light. Spectral analysis is based on Bohr's work – as light passes through an atom, the energy in the photons passes to the electrons in the outermost shell, shifting them to higher energy levels. As they return to their original position, they release the energy.

Since energy levels in the atom are discrete, from Einstein's photoelectric effect, the energy is known to produce a specific frequency of light. The atoms which make up the sun are being constantly energised to plasma, so the frequencies they would have emitted as their electrons returned to their original positions are absent from the spectrum of light the sun emits. By comparing the spectra emitted by known elements to the gaps in the sun's spectrum, it is clear that hydrogen and helium are the main elements. This question only relies on basic knowledge of vital chemical principles but requires the applicant to use these in practice. Being familiar with common experimental techniques is helpful.

Q2: You receive a small sample of a human bone of unknown age and place of origin. How might you constrain these parameters?

Hopefully, seeing the word 'age' instantly makes you think 'isotopes' - this is a question about radiometric dating and isotope fractionation. To answer the first part, you might want to start with a description of isotopes and radioactivity and write an expression for radioactive decay. But the question asks for something more – it is pushing you to explain experimentally how you determine the age. This includes choosing an appropriate isotope system (in this case Carbon has an appropriately long half-life) and describing how mass spectrometers are used to find isotopic ratios. This is a difficult question if you have no knowledge of experimental techniques, but even if you don't know the specifics, show that you understand the difference between general theory and practice.

The second part of this question, the place of origin, is a chance to show you have cross-subject knowledge or ideas even when you are out of your depth. One sample answer is to look at the ratio of Carbon-12 and Carbon-13. Recent bones from North America will contain more C-13 relative to C-12 than European bones because of the much greater use of corn. Those with biology knowledge may remember that corn is a C4 plant that takes in a higher proportion of C-13. This is just one example that shows how you can integrate your specific knowledge base into an original answer.

Q3: Which of the two molecules below is more acidic? What factors make this the case?

(A) —OH   vs.   (B)   (structure of tert-butanol with OH group)

This question is introducing the candidate to the idea that the <u>concept of acidity</u> can be applied to more molecules than just the classic "acids" you learn at school.

A good candidate would first define acidity:

$$HA \rightleftharpoons H^+ + A^-$$

Then need to <u>highlight the key reactive areas</u> on each of the molecules and assign how each of the molecules would perform when behaving as an acid. In this case, both molecules form RO- + H+ as the products. The crux of this problem is that the stability of MeO- is greater than (Me)3CO- which is because the O- is more stable in A.

Methyl groups are electron-donating groups and in molecule (B) there are three Me groups pushing onto the carbon bonded to the oxygen, therefore, this carbon is more electron-rich than molecule (A) so destabilises the O-. Consequently, the equilibrium for molecule (B) in water is more shifted towards ROH rather than RO-so molecule A is more acidic than molecule B. A good candidate will also then link this to equilibrium constants.

$$K_a = \frac{[H_3O^+]_{eq}[A^-]_{eq}}{[HA]_{eq}}$$

This question should not be too difficult - good students would be expected to give a comprehensive answer that synthesises multiple chemistry principles from the A-level syllabus. This question tests how comfortable people are with these principles and if they can use them in different scenarios.

Q4a: How do these two molecules react? Draw the mechanism.

This should be a really simple question to start with. The candidate should acknowledge the rich area of electron density in the alkene will attack a Cl atom in the symmetrical Cl-Cl causing the bond to break and form a Cl— anion.

Then the candidate needs to explain why the double bond breaks in such a way to leave the positive charge on the carbon with one Me group and one Cl atom. This is because the Me groups are electron donating, so push electron density onto that carbon and stabilise the positive charge. They also need to comment that F is more electronegative than Cl, therefore, the Cl-C bond is less polar.

The route that is normally taught in A-level is that the Cl- anion then quenches the positive charge which is then localised on that carbon and forms the product.

This, however, is not strictly the case. A standard candidate should be able to answer this question, the second part, however, will assess a standard candidate compared to a good one.

Q4b: The reaction drawn above is not complete. What else can quench that positive charge instead of the Cl? Explain the new path mechanistically.

Here the candidate should recognise that the Cl- anion is not the only nucleophile and the Cl atom in the molecule can donate a lone pair of electrons and stabilise the reactive intermediate. It forms a cyclo intermediate with the positive charge now more delocalised but, strictly speaking, primarily localised on the Cl atom. A good candidate will remark that this intermediate happens almost immediately when the carbocation is formed because intramolecular reactions happen faster than intermolecular reactions, as intermolecular reactions require a collision between the two molecules.

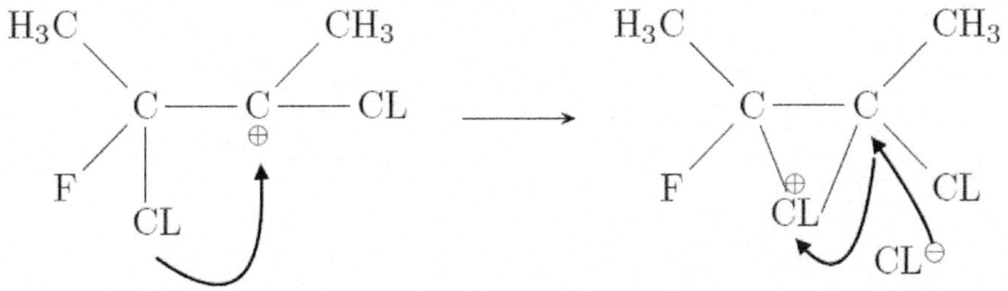

This cyclised intermediate is then attacked by the Cl- anion and relieves the steric strain of the 3 membered ring. The reaction still takes place on the same carbon because it has a lower activation energy than if the ring was opened up the other way. This forms the same product as in the original reaction mechanism. This question is a typical example of taking what a student already should know and analysing something a bit deeper.

Q5: Ketones and aldehydes in aqueous solution are typically hydrated following the mechanism below. The extent to which a ketone/aldehyde is hydrated is dominated by numerous factors. Discuss the extent of hydration of each of the molecules below and order them from most hydrated to least.

The addition of water is reversible and happens via proton transfer. The candidate should recognise the thermodynamic stability of the carbonyl versus the hydrate, which will determine the percentage of hydrate at equilibrium. This reaction is under thermodynamic control. The candidate should first discuss the percentage of hydrate for an aldehyde vs. a ketone.

Ketones are less likely to be hydrated than the equivalent aldehyde, this is because of a greater steric hindrance in molecule (B) vs. molecule (D). There is repulsion between the two Me groups as they are so close in space when the hydrate is formed as they are forced together on forming a tetrahedral hydrate. This causes the equilibrium to be towards the starting material for molecule B.

For molecule C, the candidate should acknowledge that there is a lot of strain in cyclopropanone, the $C=O$ forces the molecule to be in the same plane and the bond angles to be very small. With the addition of water to molecule (C), the steric strain is released and it can form a more stable tetrahedral molecule with an increased bond angle of $109.5°$. Therefore, the equilibrium constant for this reaction is extremely large.

For molecule (A) the candidate should comment on the effects of three Cl atoms, which are electron-withdrawing groups due to being more electronegative than C. The inductive effect of the Cl atoms increases the reactivity of the $C=O$ (a larger $\delta+$ on the C) as less electron density on neighbouring carbon atom (CCl_3) and so the water is even more strongly attracted the C in $C=O$ and therefore has a large hydration constant.

Therefore the ordering is as follows: C, A, D, B

The discussion here is more important in some respects than the ordering. But it is also testing candidates' ability to assess the dominance and importance of different factors. It would also be advisable that the candidate draws out the whole mechanism as this will show that they understand how this reaction happens and also will actually help them answer this question.

Q6: Explain mechanistically how the following reaction happens?

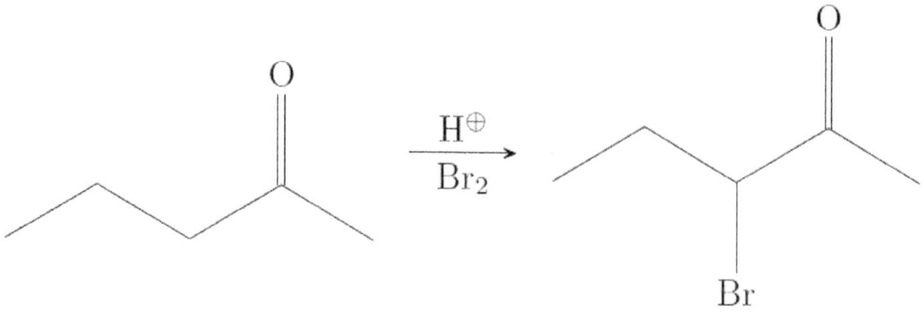

The candidate needs to analyse what will attack the acid, "H+", i.e. what is the best nucleophile in the system. The Br-Br bond is not going to break by itself so it is not that so has to be the ketone. The lone pair of electrons on the oxygen attacks the H+.

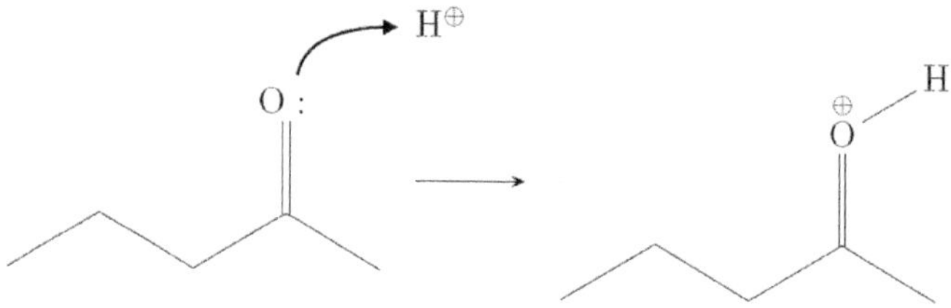

The resulting molecule can be stabilised by losing the relatively acidic proton alpha to the C=O. Thus creating an enol, ketones in acidic conditions are always in equilibrium with their enol form. The stability and where the equilibrium lies depends on the molecule. The enol form, however, can go on and actually productively react with Br2.

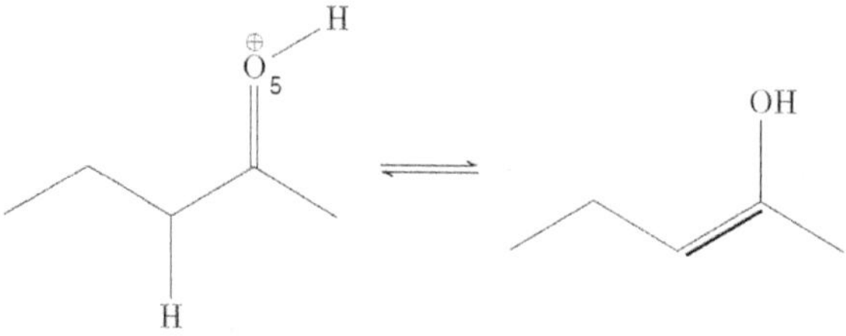

This molecule here can then attack Br-Br. Like with electrophilic addition, the electron density is going to come from the double bond and break the Br-Br sigma bond. In this instance, there is an additional driving factor; the lone pair on the oxygen can feed into the double bond and kick start the reaction with Br2.

At this point, the candidate is basically there and just needs to point out that Br- can attack the protonated ketone and form the product. This reaction step is not in equilibrium. Unlike the enolisation, once the enol has reacted with Br2 it is irreversible.

Q7: Order these atoms in decreasing first ionisation energy: Al, Ba, S, O, P and Mg.

It is first necessary to <u>define first ionisation energy</u>: $X(g)$ + e- -> $X-(g)$. The candidate should remark that O and S are both in group 16, Mg and Ba are both in group 2 Al and P are in the same row as each other as well as S and Mg. Recognition of this will help the candidate compare each of the atoms and have a nice structure.

There are two factors in this question and the candidate has to weigh them out. The first factor is that, in general, the ionisation energy across a period increases, due to an increase in effective nuclear charge. The nucleus is becoming more positively charged with the increase in protons and the outmost electrons are experiencing a similar shielding effect as they are filling up the same principal quantum number. The valence electrons are attracted more strongly and pulled in closer to the nucleus. The other factor here is that the first ionisation energy decreases as you go down a group. Although the nuclear charge increases, the valence electrons are shielded by the greater number of inner electron shells. Thus, the <u>valence electrons are further away from the nucleus</u>.

A <u>poor candidate</u> may get confused at the last point and predict that the ionisation energy increases down a group, the interviewer will check to see that they are comfortable with these two factors.

With this, you can thus conclude that O will have a higher first ionisation energy than S and Mg will have a higher first ionisation energy than Ba. Ba is last because the first ionisation energy means that a valence electron is removed from 6s orbital which is much more shielded than for Mg [He]3s² which loses an electron in 3s, [Ar]3s². You can also conclude that Mg has a lower ionisation energy than Al, [Ar] 3s²3p¹ which in turn has a lower ionisation energy than P and S, P [Ar] 3s²3p³ and S [Ar] 3s²3p⁴.

The last factor that needs to be deduced is comparing P and S. P 3p³ vs S 3p⁴. The candidate needs to recognise that whilst S has a larger <u>effective nuclear charge</u> than P, in fact, the first ionisation energy for P is larger than that of S. p energy level is comprised of 3 orbitals, p_x, p_y and p_z, Phosphorus had 3 electrons each in the three respective p orbitals, Sulphur 3p⁴ has 2 single electrons and one orbital has paired electrons. This is a less favourable electronic configuration, undergoing ionisation removes the <u>electron-electron repulsion</u> and so is rather favourable.

Q8: Draw the shapes of the following: CH4, PF5, SF6, ClF3 and SF4.

The logic for working out each of these shapes is the same. First, work out the <u>valence electrons</u> on the central atom. This tells you the area of negative charge around that atom. Then work out how many electrons each other atom gives to the central one – in single covalent bonds, it is 1 electron that is being donated. Pair the electrons up and work out the number of areas of negative charge around the atom and then this will indicate the shape of the molecule.

The first 3 molecules should be quite easy and will test to see if the candidate understands the basic principles; which can then be used to solve the latter molecules.

<u>CH₄:</u> Carbon 4 electrons, 4 x 1 e⁻ from each H. Therefore, 4 areas of negative charge, no lone pairs. So the shape is tetrahedral.

<u>PF₅:</u> P 5e⁻ , F 5 x e⁻ so 5 areas of negative charge so trigonal bipyramidal.

<u>SF₆:</u> S 6e⁻ , F 6 x e⁻ so 6 areas of negative charge so octahedral.

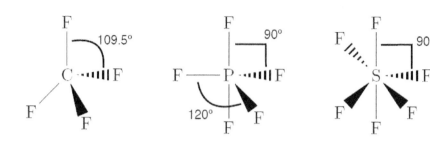

CIF_3: Cl 7e-, F 3 x e-, 5 areas of negative charge, two of which are lone pairs, so is a trigonal bipyramidal structure but lone pair–lone pair repulsion greater than bond pair–lone pair and bond pair–bond pair, therefore, the two lone pairs take up more room, creating a 't-shaped' molecule

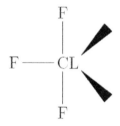

SF_4: S 6e-, F 4 x e-, so 5 areas of negative charge, this time one lone pair of electrons. A good candidate should remark that the lone pair of electrons goes in the equatorial position as it is statistically further away from all other bond paired electrons. Again this shape is based on trigonal bipyramidal but is called a "seesaw" molecular structure.

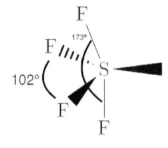

Q9: Why are metals, in particular, transition metals, coloured?

Octahedral splitting for transition metals:

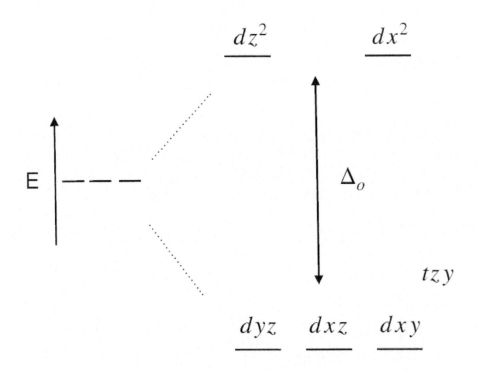

Candidates may comment on the following features:

- <u>Changes in oxidation state</u> lead to different colours - as the oxidation state changes, so do the configuration of electrons in the d-orbitals.
- The <u>absorption of white light</u> can lead to different colours. In aqueous solution, the d-orbitals split into two, but are still relatively close together. When certain wavelengths of light are absorbed, electrons in lower energy levels are excited to higher ones as they have the right energy match. The remaining photons then pass through and cause the metal to be coloured.
- The <u>shape of the molecule</u> affects the colour as it results in different electron arrangements in the d-orbitals. i.e. tetrahedral complexes are different colours to that of octahedral.

- The <u>nature of the ligand</u> itself will affect the colour – the greater the splitting of the d-orbitals, the more energy will be needed to promote electrons in the lower d-orbitals to the higher ones.

The <u>wavelength of light:</u> shorter wavelength absorption means that the colour of the complex will tend towards the blue end of the spectrum.

Q10a: Draw for me and describe a phase diagram for a hydrocarbon, pointing out key characteristics of the graph and what you can deduce from it.

A Phase diagram shows the melting, boiling and sublimation curve of a substance and also the triple point. Candidate should end up discussing all of the points highlighted below on the graph. The important thing to note is that <u>the substance is in equilibrium between gas and liquid</u>. If they do not know what one is, the examiner may draw the graph and then expect the candidate to analyse it. A question on differentiation may also be asked to calculate the melting point.

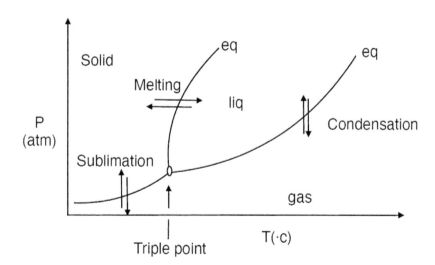

Q10b: What would this diagram look like for water?

This is slightly discussed at A-level so shouldn't be too challenging, but the phase diagram may not have been drawn before. The key thing to note is that ice takes up more volume than water (liquid), this is due to hydrogen bonding. This intermolecular force is very strong and favourable and causes the H2O molecules to align themselves in a certain arrangement so each molecule can have two hydrogen bonds each. <u>When ice melts, these hydrogen bonds are</u>

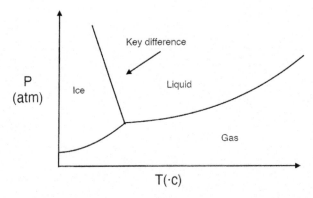

<u>broken</u> and so the water molecules can get closer together. This should then lead to the negative gradient of the melting equilibrium line.

Q11a: Describe for me what a ball in a 2D box (or well) would be like if it could only move along the x-axis and was between two infinitely high potential energy walls. Therefore, only potential energy is applicable on the ball. What would happen to the ball?

The candidate should start by drawing a potential well, drawing the y-axis and noting that it has infinite potential energy. The ball (analogy of a particle in a 1D box of Schrodinger's equation) can only move in the x-axis direction and since only potential energy is acting on the particle, it will vibrate back and forth.

Key things for candidates to note are that <u>the ball will not be able to move out of the 2D box</u>. When it approaches the y-axis, there is an infinitely large potential force acted on it and thus is repelled. Also note that the ball's potential energy would stay at the same level since no other force is acting on it.

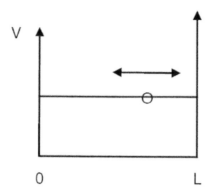

Q11b: Where is the ball statistically most likely to be found inside this potential well?

Here we are treating the ball as a particle and therefore if you label the x-axis say 0 to length L then the most probable place of finding the ball would be in the middle of the box i.e. L/2. This is applying a classic physics principle in what is a <u>quantum physics problem</u>. The ball passes through the middle the most and so is therefore most likely to be found here.

Q12: How is the solubility of a hydrocarbon affected by its double bonds?

This question presents a chance to demonstrate your knowledge of core Chemistry topics and your problem-solving skills. It is testing two things: knowledge of the factors affecting solubility and knowledge of the structure and bonding of hydrocarbons. This is an opportunity to show what you know, rather than hide what you do not know. To answer this question, we start by exploring the two factors separately and then move towards an answer.

A **good applicant**: The answer will demonstrate an understanding that solubility depends on the strength of bonding present between the solute and solvent molecules. Polar substances are soluble in polar solvents but not non-polar solvents, with the opposite true for non-polar substances. This is because polar species always prefer to interact with other polar species due to the favourable electrostatic interactions between them. Examples could be used to illustrate this point e.g., halide salts in water and saturated hydrocarbons in water:

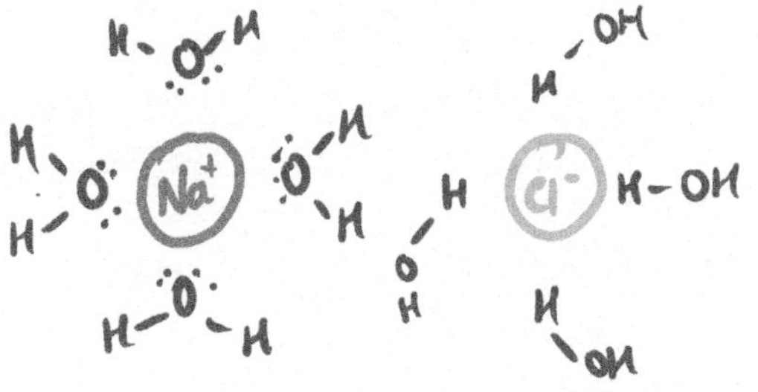

Polar water molecules interact more favourably with chlorine and sodium ions than with themselves, so NaCl is soluble in water.

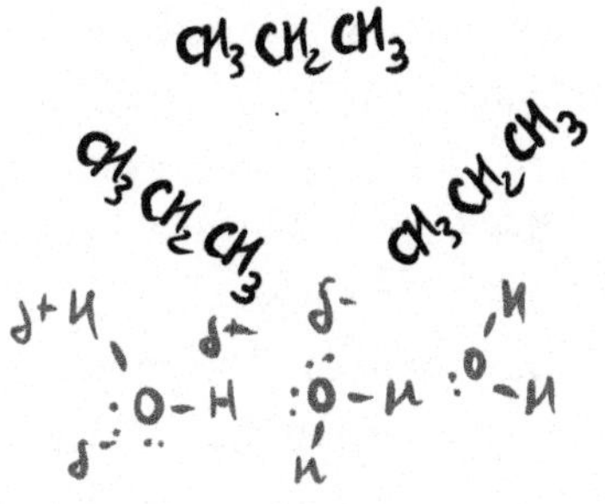

Polar water molecules have more favourable interaction with themselves than the hydrocarbon molecules, so the hydrocarbon is not soluble in water.

Then move onto exploring the bonding in hydrocarbons. The key differences between saturated (only single bonds) and unsaturated (containing double bonds) hydrocarbons are:

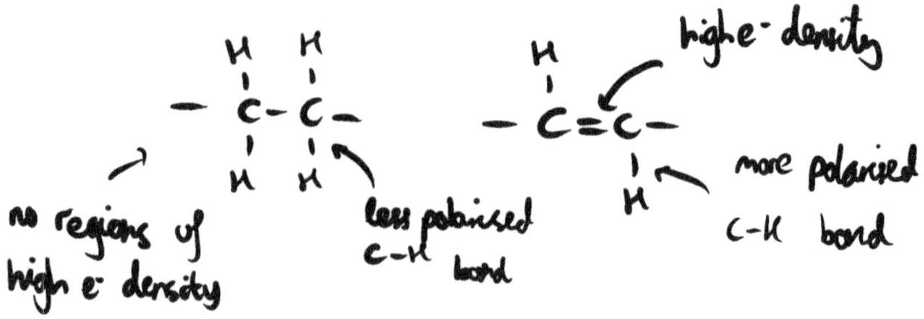

Bond polarisation could be further explored with values of electronegativity (H – 2.2, C – 2.55), whilst noting that carbon atoms attached to double bonds (sp^2) have a higher electronegativity than those with all single bonds (sp^3). However. this is quite high-level information.

Finally, explore the implications of these differences on molecule solubility e.g. unsaturated hydrocarbons are likely to have higher solubility in more polar solvents, but lower solubility in less polar solvents. The diagrams drawn throughout this answer provide an illustration of the candidate's understanding of the topic and help the candidate to think about the question more deeply.

A bad answer: This is likely a wild or educated guess. This defeats the point of this question and of the interview more broadly, which is to use your scientific knowledge to explore the problem and find a solution. Having the right final answer isn't necessarily important, but the method of getting to the answer is.

Q13: Is it possible to have an alkane with each carbon atom existing in a different environment? Can you draw it?

This is testing the interviewee on two topics, firstly their knowledge of structure and bonding of hydrocarbons and their knowledge of NMR spectroscopy.

A good answer: The answer starts with the knowledge that an alkane is an acyclic saturated hydrocarbon. To further demonstrate your knowledge, you could draw some examples:

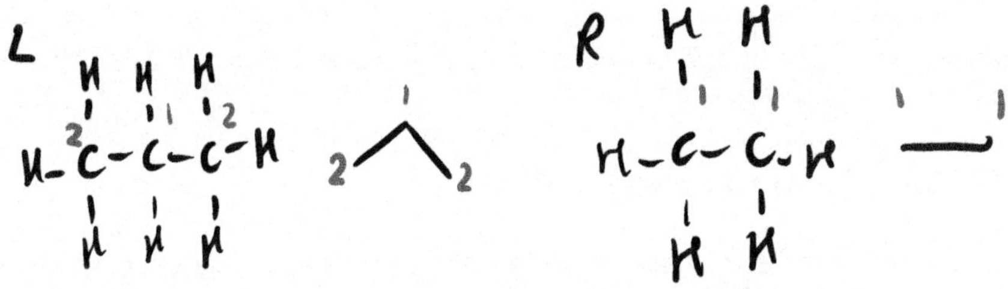

Left (L): Propane with two carbon environments. Right (R): Ethane with one carbon environment. Drawing structural and skeletal formulae help demonstrate greater chemistry knowledge.

Next, the candidate can start discussing NMR environments. Two carbon atoms have the same NMR environment if the view from both is the same, and therefore, the electron density around the nuclei will be the same. The electron density determines the strength of the induced field experienced by a given carbon nucleus in the magnetic field of the NMR machine. The induced field determines the total field felt by the carbon nucleus and hence the separation between its energy states and the frequency of energy required for resonance (i.e., the carbon nucleus to be promoted to a higher energy level). Could also note that as ^{12}C is spin-zero, ^{13}C nuclei are detected in carbon NMR. Aspects of this answer would likely arise following prompting from the interviewer/examiner, and unlikely would expect this complete answer from the start.

Above, we can see that both ethane and propane contain one less carbon environment than they do carbon atoms. This is because the end carbon atoms are in the same environment. This is true for all alkanes and so would deduce that the answer is no. Alternatively, we might suggest that methane fits the question because although it only contains one carbon environment, it also only contains one carbon atom – hence there are no two carbon atoms in the same environment. Both would be acceptable, however exploring methane is valuable as we can answer the question on a higher level.

A poor applicant may simply try to guess, make up a molecule which is not an alkane, or most commonly, give up. "I don't know how to do that is a common and very disappointing answer. If you don't know, that's okay - but ask them for help.

Q14: Describe the bonding in Al_2O_3

This question presents a chance to demonstrate your knowledge of core Chemistry topics and your problem-solving skills. It is testing one main thing in the interviewee: knowledge of structure and bonding. See this as an opportunity to show what you know, rather than hide what you don't. To answer it, we want to start by exploring this topic and move towards an answer, rather than diving in with a guess, educated or otherwise.

A good applicant: The answer will refer to the compound Al_2O_3 **containing** both a metallic element (aluminium) and a non-metallic element (oxygen), and therefore must have an ionic lattice structure. The candidate would not be expected to structure the structure of Al_2O_3 without guidance of the interviewer.

The candidate can then refer to the presence of strong ionic bonds between Al^{3+} and O^{2-} ions but there is an element of covalent bonding in the compound too due to the difference in electronegativity between Al and O. Therefore, the bonding is not purely ionic. The interviewer may then start a discussion about pure ionic and pure covalent bonding being two extremes of a spectrum, on which most compounds lie somewhere in between. Examples could be water, which is mainly covalent with some ionic component, and Al_2O_3 is mainly ionic with some covalent component.

A poor **applicant:** The answer may involve a guess what the stricture of Al_2O_3 and may not fully discussion differences in ionic and covalent bonding, or the spectrum of bonding that exists in different compounds.

Q15: How might playing in a band help you with Chemistry?

Initial reactions to this question might include thinking it is a stupid question to ask or the applicant may not have any idea how to address this question. It is intended as somewhat of an icebreaker but should still be taken seriously. For this question, the applicant can present the skills that are valuable to chemists.

A **good applicant will take** this question seriously, and highlights skills or attributes, which would make somebody a good band member. Examples include:

- Skilful with their own instrument and motivated to practice in their own time.
- Good knowledge of music theory to complement their instrumental skills.
- Ability to think creatively when making new music.
- Good team-working skills and ability to work well with other band members.
- Enthusiastic about playing their instrument and being part of the band.

Then, give examples why these skills are also useful to chemists:

- Good practical skills developed through practice.
- Good understanding of theoretical chemistry to complement laboratory.
- Thinking creatively about scientific ideas and develop new experiments.
- Effective team-worker so they can collaborate with other chemists both within their own laboratory research group and with the wider research community.
- Passionate and enthusiastic about Chemistry and are motivated to work hard.

There are many relevant skills that could be discussed beyond the list provided here.

A poor applicant: The answer fails to address with the question or makes parallels between a band member and a chemist which are not clearly relevant or discussed well. This question is designed to get you to think outside of the box, which can be difficult, but it's important to show the interviewer that you know about what being a chemist entails and show your motivations towards Chemistry.

Q16: What are the similarities and differences between ionisation energy and electronegativity?

This question is testing the interviewee in two main ways: their knowledge of structure and bonding and their knowledge of thermodynamics.

A good applicant: First, the answer should provide definitions of the key terms mentioned in the question. *Electronegativity:* the tendency of an atom to attract electrons in a bond towards it. *Ionisation energy:* the energy required to remove an electron from one mole of atoms. For ionisation energy, a diagram might be useful (M represents any element):

$$M_{(g)} \longrightarrow M^+_{(g)} + e^-$$

The next step would be to discuss similarities and differences between the two terms. Firstly, their similarities:

- Both are a measure of the strength of bonding between the nucleus of an atom and the electrons in its outer shell.
- Both are affected by the shielding of outer shell electrons by electrons, which lie between the outer shell and the nucleus.
- Both are dependent upon the effective nuclear charge (Z_{eff}) experienced by outer shell electrons.
- The trends of ionisation energy and electronegativity on the periodic table are generally the same.

Next, the differences between the two:

- They don't show the same trends across periods 2 and 3. Ionisation energies show a characteristic dip at B and Al as the p-orbitals begin to be filled and then at O and S when electrons begin to be paired in p-orbitals. However, for electronegativity we see a monotonical increase across both periods.
- Electronegativity is not an exact quantity in the same way that ionisation energy is. There is no one measurement we can do to determine the electronegativity of an element.

There are a number of further, more detailed points which could be made, but these are well beyond the scope of knowledge expected of an A-level student. The latter points about the differences between the two are likely to be prompted by an interviewer.

A poor applicant does not know the definitions of these two terms (basic knowledge at A-level) or does not properly discuss their similarities and differences.

Q17: What makes life carbon based? Why not silicon?

This question is testing the interviewee's knowledge of organic chemistry and their knowledge of biological chemistry. To answer this question, start by exploring the relevant properties of carbon and contrast those with the relevant properties of silicon.

A good applicant starts the answer by exploring the attributes of carbon that make it suitable as a foundation for life on earth:

- High valency: Each carbon atom can form up to four bonds, with a wide range of different elements, which can be either stable e.g., C-H or reactive e.g., C=O.
- Versatility: Carbon can form molecules with a variety of different shapes e.g., long and short-chain linear molecules including polymers (both addition and condensation), planar and non-planar rings. The carbon atoms in these structures can have bonds in tetrahedral, trigonal, or linear arrangements — as in alkanes, alkenes and alkynes respectively.

- Availability: When carbon is oxidised a gas (CO_2) is generated, which is accessible for plants

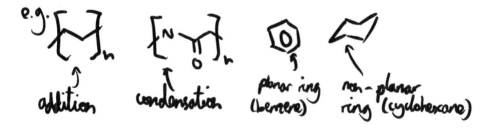

Now, the applicant should compare carbon with silicon:

- High valency: Silicon can also form four bonds, however, many of these are not stable (in part due to the larger size of silicon atoms, meaning it struggles to fit four bonds around itself)
- Versatility: Less versatile than carbon but can still form polymers and bond to oxygen.

- Availability: When silicon is oxidised, it forms a solid – SiO_2 – i.e., sand, which would be much harder for theoretical Si-based plants to absorb and use.

e.g. $\left[O \diagdown \underset{\displaystyle |}{\overset{\displaystyle R}{Si}} {}^{\cdots R} \right]_n$ ← Si & O backbone

There are several other comparisons that could be explored, but these are a good foundation for the answer.

A poor applicant may get flustered by this question. This is unhelpful, especially given how difficult the question is – the struggle is not down to bad preparation on the part of the applicant. The candidate may also refer to properties of carbon that are not relevant e.g., that carbon forms allotropes such as diamond and graphite.

Q18: If the nucleus and electrons are oppositely charged, why aren't the electrons sufficiently attracted to the nucleus to crash into it?

This question is testing knowledge of the structure of an atom.

A good applicant explains the Bohr model of the atom:
- Positively charged nucleus at the centre of the atom. The nucleus contains positively charged protons and neutrally charged neutrons. The existence of the nucleus was discovered by Rutherford in experiments where he fired alpha particles at a thin gold foil. Subsequently, neutrons were discovered by Chadwick when he fired alpha radiation at Beryllium and the neutrally charged particles (neutrons) generated were subsequently fired at paraffin.
- Negatively charged electrons exist in discrete (fixed) energy levels around this nucleus. E.g. 1s, 2s, 2p, 3s, 3p, 4s, 3d etc. in order of ascending energy. The electron was discovered by J.J. Thomson using cathode rays, and the energy levels were discovered by Bohr using evidence such as emission and absorption spectra of different gases.

The quantised energy levels discovered by Bohr prevents the electrons from falling into the nucleus. These are a product of quantum mechanics, which is a description of nature on an atomic level. This differs from the description of nature we have on a macroscopic scale –classical mechanics. The hallmark of quantum mechanics is the presence of "quantised" energy levels i.e. that quantum systems – like the atom – have discrete energy states and that these energy states correspond to fixed values of energy. This is in contrast to macroscopic systems e.g. orbiting planets, which have a continuous range of energy states depending on the distance between them.

In a classical picture of the atom, we would expect electrons to fall into the nucleus. This is because as they orbit the nucleus, we would expect them to emit electromagnetic radiation and so lose kinetic energy and hence speed. The slower the electron travels, the closer it must orbit the nucleus and eventually it would crash into it. This was a key issue with the model of the atom before Bohr, as it's not what we observe. However, in the quantum mechanical picture we have something quite different. The electron is viewed not as a particle but as something with a mixture of wave-like and particle properties. It is described by a wavefunction, which describes the probability of an electron being in a given position at a given time. Because the electron is not in an "orbit" – it does not move in circular motion around the nucleus - it does not emit electromagnetic radiation and so the energy of an atom will remain constant (provided the atom is isolated from radiation, which it could absorb). If the electron moves closer to the nucleus it will convert potential energy to kinetic energy, without the total energy of the atom ever changing. It can never reach the nucleus because this would require the electron to gain infinite kinetic energy, as when two like charges have no distance between them their potential energy is negatively infinite.

A poor applicant fails to recall the structure of the atom including quantised energy levels. These quantised nature of energy levels should be second nature to any Physical Natural Sciences candidate, and they are key to solving this question. Equally, engaging with the discussion around why quantised energy levels solve this problem constructively is a must.

Q19: What is the significance of the bonding in benzene?

This question is testing the interviewee's knowledge of the structure and bonding of benzene.

A good candidate begins by exploring the structure and bonding in benzene. A good place to start is experimental evidence for benzene's unusual structure. It was previously thought that benzene had 3 C=C double bonds (Kekule structure/1,3,5-cyclohexatriene) but there were issues with this:

- All 6 C-C distances in benzene were equal.
- Benzene did not undergo the usual addition reactions that you would predict from an alkene.
- The enthalpy of hydrogenation is much less negative than expected (by 152 kJ mol^{-1}) suggesting the true structure is significantly more stable (stronger bonding) than the Kekule structure.

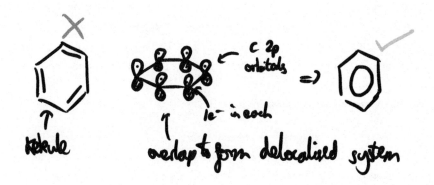

As drawn above, benzene's true structure contains six carbon 2p orbitals that overlap to form a delocalised system of π orbitals. A good applicant might also mention that the carbon atoms in this structure are sp^2 hybridised, giving the benzene molecule its planar shape (which would also be true for the hypothetical 1,3,5 – cyclohexatriene). This is a much more stable bonding arrangement than the three double bonds in Kekule's structure and which explains the issues above:

- There is equal electron density between all C atoms, so all bonds have equal lengths.
- This structure does not undergo the usual addition reactions because the stable delocalised system would need to be broken (requiring roughly 150 kJ mol^{-1}).
- The less negative hydrogenation enthalpy is also explained by more stable bonding.

The "significance" of this bonding is that it shows a delocalised, rather than localised, picture of bonding in a molecule. Six electrons are shared between six atoms, rather than two electrons between two atoms, as in conventional sigma or pi covalent bonds. The interviewer might also explore how this bonding contributes to the "ring current" phenomenon observed in NMR spectra of benzene and its derivatives.

A poor applicant fails to remember the structure of benzene, or why it is unusual. It isn't necessary to remember everything mentioned above (particularly not values for stability etc.) but knowing that all six carbon 2p orbitals overlap to give a delocalised bonding regime would be expected.

Q20: How do you synthesise aspirin?

This is a question designed to test a mixture of practical and theoretical Chemistry knowledge. It is looking to explore a specific organic synthesis, which the applicant is likely to have come across before (it is on the A-Level specification). For this question, it is not necessarily important to get the details perfect, and the precise equipment is not important but it's important to have thorough reasoning for everything you discuss.

A good applicant begins their answer with the structures of the starting material (salicylic acid) and the product (aspirin). You would not be expected to produce complete diagrams from memory:

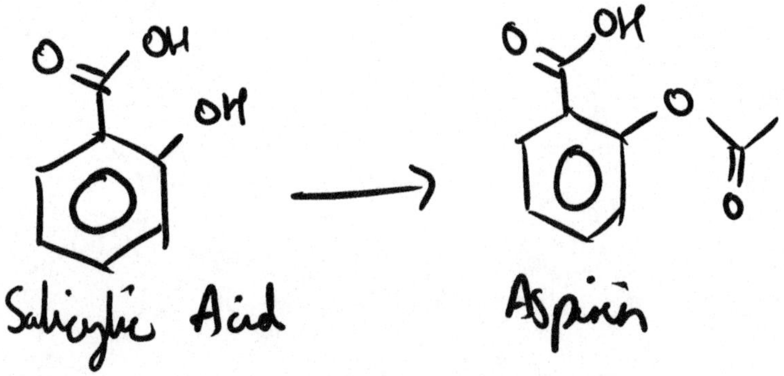

Note that the only part of the structure, which has changed is the OH group attached to the benzene ring in salicylic acid, hence it must be involved in the mechanism. Since the OH group is nucleophilic (due to its two lone pairs), the mechanism is likely to be a nucleophilic substitution on a carbonyl compound. There are two possible carbonyl compounds which could be used: ethanoyl chloride and ethanoic anhydride. The interviewer might ask you to explore why ethanoic anhydride is used in industry:

- Ethanoic anhydride is cheaper than ethanoyl chloride.
- Ethanoic anhydride is safer to use as HCl is not produced, which is corrosive and poisonous.
- Ethanoic anhydride is less reactive so is hydrolysed less easily.

If asked to suggest a catalyst, sulfuric and phosphoric are both options. This is useful because it makes ethanoic anhydride more reactive, by increasing the partial positive charge on the carbonyl carbon atom.

The mechanism for the reaction could also be drawn:

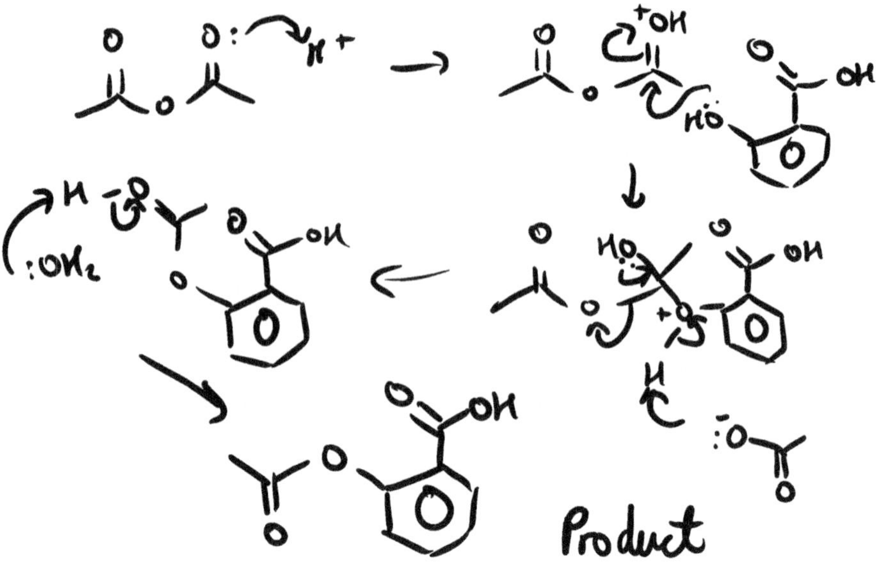

The applicant could also mention that the by-product is ethanoic acid and that the acid is regenerated in the reaction. The process of how to carry out these steps in a laboratory may or may not then be explored by with interviewer. The key steps are:

- React the salicylic acid and ethanoic anhydride, together with the acid catalyst, in a flask submerged in a water bath at roughly 75°C.
- After 15 minutes or so add water to hydrolyse any remaining ethanoic anhydride.
- Cool using ice bath until aspirin has fully crystallised and remove using a Büchner funnel.
- Dissolve the aspirin collected in warm ethanol and complete a recrystallisation to remove any residual ethanoic acid.

The interviewer might ask you to explore why each step is carried out in the way it is to test your knowledge of the process.

A poor applicant does not apply their knowledge to deduce that the mechanism must be a nucleophilic substitution or fails to suggest a relevant and plausible mechanism. The mechanism does not need to be perfect but the two key steps should be correct: these are the nucleophilic attack by OH and ethanoate ion leaving anhydride (or Cl leaving ethanoyl chloride if this is reactant used). This question is requires you to demonstrate your knowledge of an important reaction type in organic chemistry and its mechanism.

Q21: How would you distinguish diamond from graphite?

This question is testing the interviewee's knowledge of the structure, bonding and properties of carbon allotropes.

A good applicant starts their answer by explaining that diamond and graphite are two allotropes of carbon i.e., that they are both pure forms of carbon in which the atoms bond to each other in different ways, producing a different structure with different properties. Starting with the structure, bonding, and properties of diamond:

- Each C atom is sp^3 hybridised and makes 4 single covalent bonds to other C atoms and these bonds are tetrahedrally arranged.
- These strong covalent bonds extend throughout diamond's macromolecular structure and in all directions – giving it a high strength, melting and boiling point, as well as high thermal conductivity.
- Diamond's structure has no free electrons (they are all localised in the covalent bonds) and so diamond is a poor conductor of electricity.

Then moving onto the structure, bonding, and properties of graphite:

- Each C atom is sp^2 hybridised, making 3 single bonds each to other C atoms. These bonds have a trigonal arrangement and extend out to form a 2-dimensional hexagonal lattice.
- Each C atom has a lone 2p orbital containing one electron, and these 2p orbitals overlap to form a huge delocalised orbital system.
- These delocalised electrons result in graphite being a good conductor of electricity.
- However, there are no covalent bonds between the hexagonal layers, only weak Van der Waals forces, hence graphite is weak, and the layers slide easily over one another.

- The strong covalent bonds present within the layers give graphite a high thermal conductivity although it is less than that of diamond.

The interviewer might then discuss how graphene, another allotrope of carbon, is different from graphite and diamond, or discuss the allotropes of other elements such as phosphorous.

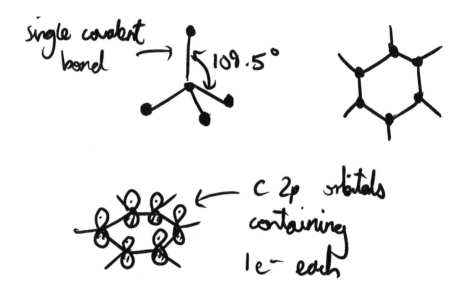

A poor applicant lacks knowledge about graphite and diamond such as the fact they are allotropes of carbon, or how their structure and bonding affect key properties such as electrical conductivity. These topics should be well understood by any applicant.

Q22: What underpins Le Chatelier's principle?

This question is testing the interviewee's knowledge of thermodynamics.

A good applicant begins by defining Le Chatelier's principle:

"When a change in temperature, pressure, volume or concentration is imposed on a system in dynamic equilibrium, the position of that equilibrium will move and in such a way as to oppose the change"

The applicant will then discuss the principle further:

- Dynamic equilibrium is a state in which both forward and reactions are occurring at the same time. The exact rate of each reaction is the same so that the concentrations of all reactants and products remain constant.
- If the temperature is increased, the endothermic reaction would be favoured so that the system absorbs heat. This decreases the temperature of the system.
- If the concentration of a product was decreased (e.g. a gas evaporates), then the forward reaction would be favoured to increase the concentration of that product.

The applicant might discuss specific examples of reactions in their answer such as the Haber process:

$$3H_{2(g)} + N_{2(g)} \underset{\text{backward}}{\overset{\text{forward}}{\rightleftharpoons}} 2NH_{3(g)}$$

There are more gaseous moles n the left hand side of the reaction, so if you increase the pressure of the system, then by Le Chatelier's principle, the forward direction would be then favoured. This would lead to a decrease in the number of gas moles and reduce the pressure.

Then the applicant can discuss the reasoning behind Le Chatelier's principle. The two cases which it's possible to explain simply are for changes in concentration and changes in pressure. The key here is that the equilibrium constant (both K_c and K_p) for a reaction depends only on temperature — changes in volume, pressure or concentration won't affect its value. Thinking about changes in concentration using Haber process:

- If ammonia is removed its concentration will decrease.
- For K_c to stay the same, more ammonia must be produced so that its concentration increases and those of hydrogen and nitrogen decrease.
- This is the change that will keep K_c constant and follows Le Chatelier's principle.

$$k_c = \frac{[NH_3]^2}{[H_2]^3[N_2]}$$

Thinking about changes in pressure using Haber process:

- If the pressure is increased, K_p will decrease.
- The mole fraction of ammonia must be increased by favouring the forward reaction, as predicted by Le Chatelier's principle.

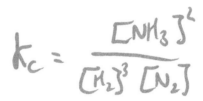

$$k_p = \frac{p_{NH_3}^2}{p_{H_2}^3 \, p_{N_2}} = \frac{x_{NH_3}^2}{x_{H_2}^3 \, x_{N_2} \, p^2} \qquad x \text{ is mole fraction} \\ P \text{ is total pressure}$$

The explanation in terms of volume can be taken as the converse of that for pressure – pV is constant for isothermal systems – whilst the explanation in terms of temperature is much trickier and would not be expected from an applicant, although the interviewer might walk you through it.

A poor applicant fails to recall Le Chatelier's principle, even though it should be familiar. The explanation for Le Chatelier's principle is tricky and would not be expected without prompting from the interviewer but knowing and explaining the principle itself is vital to answer this question well.

Q23: What does pH stand for?

This question is testing the interviewee's knowledge of acid and base theory.

A good applicant starts by defining pH:

$$pH = -\log_{10}([H^+]) \quad \text{where } [H^+] \text{ in mol dm}^{-3}$$

Then the applicant can give examples of how this definition would be applied. For example, a neutral solution with pH 7 has a concentration of protons measured at 10^{-7} mol dm^{-3}. The applicant might note that the 'p' in pH is a shorthand way of representing the negative base-10 logarithm of a quantity, in this case the concentration of protons (or more accurately hydroxonium ions) which are represented by a H.

The applicant may also refer to the misleading nature of using [H$^+$] since free protons do not exist in solution. In fact the species whose concentration we are measuring is the hydroxonium ion H$_3$O$^+$ (again with concentration in mol dm^{-3}):

$$pH = -\log_{10}([H_3O^+]) \qquad H\!-\!\overset{..}{\underset{H}{O}}\!^{+}\!\cdots H \quad \text{is its structure}$$

A poor applicant fails to provide a definition of pH and to engage in the subsequent discussion around the strength of an acid. Both of these areas should come easily to applicants as they form a core part of the Chemistry syllabus.

Q24: What would you say was the total mass of O2 in this building?

This is a question designed to test your ability to think outside the box and apply your Chemistry knowledge in unfamiliar questions. As an estimation question it isn't the answer which matters, but the reasoning – so don't jump in.

A **good applicant** recognises that the ideal gas law will be useful, and estimates the parameters within it:

$$pV = nRT$$

$$n = \frac{pV}{RT}$$

$$p = 100 \text{ kPa (atmospheric)}$$

$$V = ? \ m^3$$

$$R = 8.31 \ J \ mol^{-1} \ k^{-1}$$

$$T = 20°C = 293 \ k$$

Knowing that atmospheric pressure is roughly 100 kPa is useful and you can estimate the room temperature of 20°C. The most interesting calculation is probably the volume, which will depend on the building in which you are sat. A simple estimate would be to assume your building was a regular prism – cuboid, cylinder, triangular prism – or a composite of different regular prisms. To refine this estimate, you then might estimate the volume removed from the building by the walls and the other items in different rooms/areas, as none of this can be occupied by air. Once you have arrived at a reasonable estimate of the volume then calculate the number of moles of gas we expect, multiply that by the proportion of the air which is oxygen (20.95% - 20% would be fine) and then by the relative molecular mass of an oxygen molecule (approx. 32 g mol^{-1}).

For example, with a volume of 55.6 m³, pressure of 100 kPa and temperature of 300K, we get 2230 moles of gas. Hence roughly 450 moles of oxygen which has a mass of 14 kg. However, the interviewer is more interested in your methodology and not the exact value of your answer.

Qualitative refinements to this estimate you could mention are:

- How well ventilated the rooms in the building are, as poorly ventilated rooms will have lower than atmospheric oxygen concentrations due to respiration.
- Account for any plants in the room that will be producing oxygen.
- Use a law more accurate than the ideal gas law, which contains a lot of assumptions (but you would not be expected to know such a law).
- Anything else you can think of – be creative! – that is the point of this question.

A poor applicant does not recognise that the ideal gas equation would be useful. This is a key equation for chemists and similar questions may have been used regularly throughout the applicant's chemistry education. To estimate the mass of gas we need an equation to find the moles of that gas – for which the ideal gas equation should suggest itself. Also, engaging in the discussion about refining your model is key for an estimation question as you want your estimate to be as good as possible. Show off your problem-solving skills!

Q25: What makes an acid strong or weak?

This question is testing the interviewee's knowledge of acid and base theory.

A good applicant correctly recognises that strong and weak acids are distinguished by the extent to which they dissociate when added to water. A typical acid (HA) exists in equilibrium and its conjugate base (A⁻) in solution with water:

$$HA + H_2O \rightleftharpoons A^- + H_3O^+$$

The extent to which this equilibrium is shifted to the right determines the strength of the acid. Generally, the term strong acid refers to acids for which the equilibrium is so far right that the acid can be considered completely dissociated (i.e., no HA molecules exist). In contrast, weak acids refer to all others i.e. acids existing in some kind of equilibrium. The applicant can then give examples of each type of acid, for example, HCl is a strong acid and ethanoic acid is a weak acid.

The applicant may then refer to the dissociation constant, K_a, and its sister measurement, pKa, as quantitative measurements of the strength of an acid:

$$k_a = \frac{[A^-][H_3O^+]}{[HA]} \qquad pk_a = -\log_{10}[k_a]$$

It might additionally be noted that water is omitted from the equation for K_a because there is so little acid present that the concentration of water can be considered constant and hence ignored. Therefore, K_a is *not* an equilibrium constant for this dissociation, but the equilibrium constant multiplied by the concentration of water.

A poor applicant does not recall the definition of strong and weak acids or tries to use pH as a measure of the acid strength. pH measures the concentration of hydroxonium ions, but as this depends on the moles of acid added to the solution then it can't be used as a measurement of acid strength.

Q26. What's your favourite element?

This is a good icebreaking question that is used to assess your level of interest in Chemistry and your motivations behind studying Chemistry. Here it is important to be thoughtful as to what you select and to provide good reasoning – there is no right answer but the interviewer will be testing your reasoning and discussion.

A good applicant chooses an element that is either their favourite, or an element that they like for a particular reason. A few examples of possible answers are:

- Iron: It is the element with the most stable nucleus and one which is a building block of modern civilisation. As a transition metal its variable oxidation states are used in catalysing the reduction of molecular oxygen to water (it goes from Fe(II) to Fe(IV)), in our bodies. We find iron everywhere from bridges to battleships, from cutlery to breakfast cereal. Also, my favourite sculpture – the angel of the North – was made from steel (an alloy whose main constituent element is iron).

- Silicon: Silicon is one of the two elements present in silicon dioxide, the macromolecular structure, which is the main constituent of sand, and forms the basis for many common glasses. Silicon is also vital for the electronics – my phone, laptop etc. – which are so important to modern life. Due to its semiconducting electronic structure, it is used in ubiquitous components called transistors.

- Nitrogen: Nitrogen is the main component of the air we breathe, although it is so inert that it does not interact with us at all. It is also present in the nitrates that are absorbed by plant roots and is used to form other important molecules.

This is not an exhaustive list and can be expanded on by each candidate. But this does give you a good guideline on the types of things you may discuss. The key is to show you are passionate about with the element you have chosen and you are able to display your knowledge/passion for Chemistry.

A poor applicant spends a long time thinking about which specific element to choose, or says they do not have one. Equally, using bad reasoning would be undesirable as it does not show your knowledge of Chemistry.

- Gold: It is worth a lot of money.
- Lead: It is poisonous.

Q27: What's the cause of the vibrant colours in transition metals?

This question is testing the interviewee's knowledge of transition metal theory. Note that this is the kind of question that is likely to be developed upon further by the interviewer, so be prepared for unfamiliar content and further discussion.

A good applicant begins their answer by explaining what a transition metal is. Transition metals are elements that form one or more stable ions with a partially filled d-shell. The applicant may give examples such as Fe^{2+} or Cu^{2+}. The applicant may recall that transition metals are characterised by variable oxidation states, they are good catalysts and form colourful complexes. If applicant may give specific examples of colours of some common transition metal complexes (e.g. hexa-aqua or hexa-ammonia ions) to show their knowledge of the topic:

$$[Co(H_2O)_6]^{2+} \rightarrow$$

(structure drawing of hexa-aqua complex) $^{2+}$ is **RED**

$$[Cr(NH_3)_6]^{2+} \rightarrow$$

(structure drawing of hexa-ammonia complex) $^{2+}$ is **PURPLE**

The applicant can then explain why these complexes are coloured. As with any coloured object, transition metal complexes appear a certain colour because they absorb a specific wavelength of visible light. The colour the transition metal complex appears is the complement of the coloured light that it absorbs. For example, if the complex absorbs blue light it will appear yellow and if the complex absorbs red light it will appear cyan.

The applicant can then specify that a specific wavelength is absorbed when an electron in the complex is promoted between two discrete energy levels. These energy levels correspond to the d-orbitals of
the metal atom/ion. With prompting from the interviewer, the applicant might then draw the energy levels produced when a transition metal ion is coordinated octahedrally by 6 ligands. This would not be expected to be produced without guidance from the interviewer and might then lead to a discussion of the factors which might affect the energy gap (ΔE) and hence the colour a complex appears.

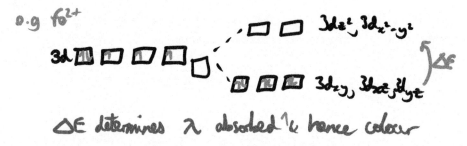

A poor applicant may incorrectly remember the definition or properties of transition metal ions and their complexes. This is expected knowledge for applicants and should be recalled with ease. The latter part of the discussion, around the specific form of the orbitals relevant to the coloured nature of these complexes, whilst not expected knowledge, should be engaged with properly.

Q28: Here's a pen - on the whiteboard, can you draw all of the isomers of C_4H_8?

This question is designed to test your knowledge of core Chemistry topics and ability to apply them to a scenario that should be reasonably familiar. The main thing this aims to test in applicants is their organic chemistry knowledge, specifically on isomers.

A good applicant refers to different types of isomerism: structural isomerism and stereoisomerism and then explain them. Structural isomerism is when the bonds are between different atoms and stereoisomerism is where the bonds are between the same atoms, but the spatial arrangement of those atoms is different. The applicant can then state there are three types of structural isomerism – chain, positional, functional – and two types of stereoisomerism – geometric and optical. They may also briefly explain these different sub-types.

The applicant can then refer to what possible functional groups a species with this molecular formula (C_4H_8) might have: alkene or cyclic alkane. Then, the applicant can draw the skeletal/structural formulae:

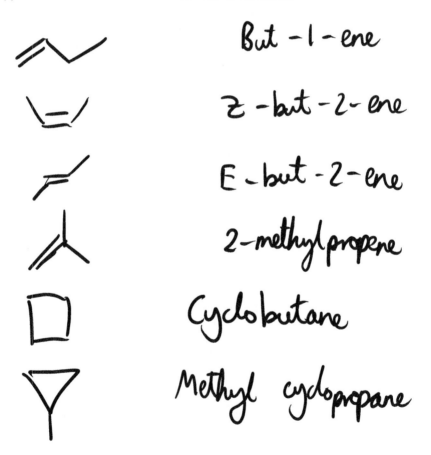

But –1–ene

Z –but –2–ene

E –but –2–ene

2–methylpropene

Cyclobutane

Methyl cyclopropane

Recognising the different types of isomerism is key here: but-1-ene and but-2-ene are positional isomers, E and Z-but-2-ene are geometric isomers (due to restricted rotation about the C=C, π bond). The alkenes and the cycloalkanes are functional isomers and 2-methylpropene and methylcyclopropane are chain isomers of butene and cyclobutene respectively. There are no optical isomers possible with this molecular formula. This is all of the possible isomers. The applicant should recognise they have finished when they have explored all the different forms of isomerism.

A poor applicant fails to recall the different types of isomerism or to explore the options for isomerism fully. The interviewer knows you won't be able to pluck the 6 isomers above out of thin air but would expect a good fundamental knowledge of isomerism and the ability to apply this knowledge to solve the problem given.

Q29: How would you go about calculating the number of moles of water in this bottle?

This is an estimation question, designed to test your ability to think outside the box and apply your Chemistry knowledge in unfamiliar questions. As an estimation question there is not one answer but it is the reasoning and methodology that is important.

A good applicant recognises that the formula Mass = M_r x moles can be used to answer this question. The mass of water in the bottle is required and so we need volume and density. The volume is unlikely to be written on the side of the bottle so we should estimate its volume by assuming the bottle to be a regular cylinder, or perhaps a composite of a cuboid and a pyramid, depending on the shape of the bottle:

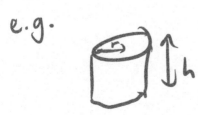

Here, it is not important to know the formulae and the interviewer may prompt you with them. The interviewer is more interested in your methodology to approximate the answer. Once you know the volume of water, you should know its density is 1.00 g cm^{-3} and use this to calculate its mass. Then use an M_r of 18 g mol^{-1} to find the number of moles using the Mass $= M_r$ x moles equation.

$$V = \pi r^2 h \qquad \text{(with cylinder)}$$

$$\text{mass} = \rho V = \pi \rho r^2 h$$

$$\text{moles} = \text{mass} / M_r = \frac{\pi \rho r^2 h}{18}$$

The model could be refined qualitatively:

- Noting that all the volume in the bottle might not be water because there may be metal ions (such as Ca^{2+} and Mg^{2+}) or microplastic particles may also be contained within the bottle.
- Estimate the quantity of metal ions from knowledge of hardness of local water or from an experiment such as titrating soap into samples of the water

A poor applicant does not recognise the usefulness of the formula Mass $= M_r$ x moles or engage properly with refining the model used for estimation. With estimation questions, recognising a method and then refining that method are the two key steps – do not worry about getting the right answer.

Q30: Why do we make catalysts from transition metals?

This question aims to test an applicant on their inorganic chemistry knowledge, specifically about transition metals.

A good applicant begins their answer by stating their knowledge of the transition metals: they are elements that form one or more stable ions with a partially filled d-shell, have variable oxidation states and can form a variety of different complexes, which are often coloured. Examples could be given to illustrate these points:

$$Cr(H_2O)_6^{3+} \quad \text{is purple} \quad Cr^{3+}: [Ar]\ 3d^3$$

$$Cr(OH)_6^{3-} \quad \text{is green} \quad Cr^{3+}: [Ar]\ 3d^3$$

$$Cr_2O_7^{2-} \quad \text{is orange} \quad Cr(IV): [Ar]$$

$$CrO_4^{2-} \quad \text{is yellow} \quad Cr(IV): [Ar]$$

The applicant then explores why these properties might make a transition metal a good catalysts:

- Variable oxidation states allow transition metals to be oxidised or reduced and make them versatile catalysts.
- Their ability to coordinate bonds with a variety of different ligands, so ligand exchange reactions can take place easily e.g., a reactant could join a complex and a product be displaced.

The coloured nature of transition metals is not relevant and having partially filled d-shells is only relevant because it is the property giving them variable oxidation states. Partially filled d-shells reveals that the outer electrons are in d-orbitals, which are well shielded so these electrons can be lost or gained easily i.e. the ions can be reduced or oxidised easily.

For this latter section of this question, the interviewer might present a specific example of a catalysis reaction which uses a transition metal such as polymerisation or hydrogenation. The interviewer may give prompts and walk through the question and discussion with the applicant in order to make clear the connection between the properties of transition metals and their usefulness as catalysts. There would not be an expectation for applicants to know these reasons already, only to show good reasoning skills and approach the problem with curiosity.

A poor applicant fails to recall the key properties of transition metals, in particular variable oxidation states and their ability to form complexes with a range of different ligands. These are the properties relevant to this question.

Q31: How do you think the density of air in the room differs from that outside? How does it differ from the air in Beijing?

This is another example of an estimation question and is designed to test your ability to think outside the box and apply your Chemistry knowledge to an unfamiliar question. Again, the exact answer is not important rather the reasoning.

A good applicant recognises that we need the mass and the volume of the gas to calculate its density, and that the ideal gas law and Mass = M_r x moles equation will be necessary to find these quantities. Then, the applicant derives an equation for the density of a gas in terms of its M_r, temperature, pressure, and the ideal gas constant, as below:

$$① \quad pV = nRT \quad ② \quad m = Mr \times n$$

$$pV = \frac{m}{Mr} \cdot RT \quad \Rightarrow \quad \frac{m}{V} = \frac{\rho Mr}{RT}$$

$$= \frac{\rho Mr}{RT}$$

i.e. ρ (density)

Now, the applicant will find the solution to M_r, pressure and temperature of the air and thinking about how they may vary between the room, the outside and in Beijing. Tackle each part in turn:

- The M_r should be the (mean) average molecular mass of the different constituent molecules in air. A first approximation could be to take it as the M_r of nitrogen gas (the most abundant element in the air at roughly 79%), then to include oxygen (roughly 20%) and then trace other gases such as carbon dioxide, argon etc. Including these trace gases might be interesting, as they show the power of estimation by having very little effect on the value obtained for density.

- The applicant may then reflect how there may be less oxygen and more carbon dioxide indoors than outdoors due to respiration, but that the composition of the air is not likely to change between here and Beijing. However, the applicant could discuss that Beijing may have increased air pollution.

- The temperature is likely to be warmer indoors (although on a hot day air conditioning may counteract this) and temperature likely to be different between here and Beijing.

- The pressure (100 kPa atmospheric pressure) will be the same across these 3 locations

Whilst thinking about these different factors and how best to approach them in each case, the applicant is likely to be asked to do a range of calculations for different levels of refinement and perhaps to come up with a final value for each three of the locations. However, as an estimation question, the values in themselves are not important but the reasoning with which the values are reached is.

A poor applicant does not recall the correct formulae and fails to engage in the discussion about refining the model for estimation. As ever with estimation, refining the model is key because it allows us to get closer to the true answer.

Q32: How would you distinguish between entropy and enthalpy?

A good applicant starts by defining and explaining entropy and enthalpy:

- Entropy is the measure of the amount of disorder in a system. For example, when a solid melts or a liquid boils, the amount of disorder, and hence the entropy of that system, increases. The applicant may also mention the second law of thermodynamics.
- Enthalpy is a quantity linked closely to the internal energy of a system (H = U + pV where U is the internal energy, p is the pressure and V is the volume – the pV term is the work done to establish the system's dimensions). Enthalpy measures the total energy – both kinetic and potential – of a system. When a solid melts or a liquid boils, the internal energy increases (bonds are weakened, so potential energy increases and particles move more, so kinetic energy increases) and hence enthalpy increases.

Entropy and enthalpy are fundamentally different quantities, while entropy measures the disorder of a system enthalpy measures the energy of a system. These two, however, are combined when we think about the Gibbs energy of a system (G = H + TS) or the change in Gibbs energy during a process:

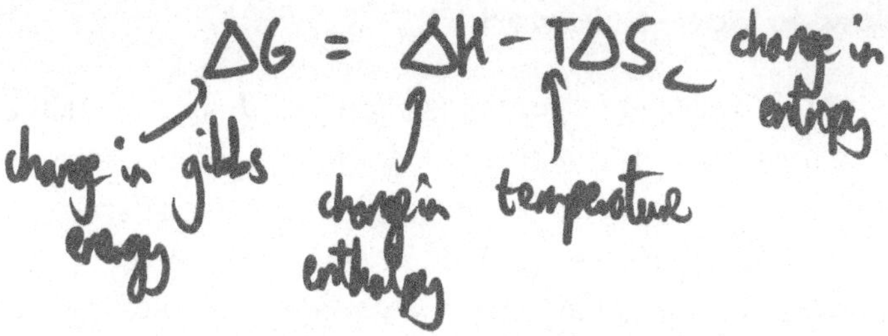

$$\Delta G = \Delta H - T\Delta S$$

change in gibbs energy

change in temperature

enthalpy

change in entropy

The interviewer might then explore Gibbs energy further by noting that a change in ΔG must be less than zero for a spontaneous process and how this is a restatement of the second law of thermodynamics given above, however this would not be expected from the applicant. The applicant might then use the knowledge that $\Delta G = 0$ for a system in equilibrium, and apply the statements made above:

• When solids melt at their melting point, $\Delta G = 0$, which fits with our qualitative understanding that both the enthalpy and entropy should increase during this process.

• When liquids boil at their boiling point, $\Delta G = 0$, which fits with our qualitative understanding that both the enthalpy and entropy should increase during this process.

Note that it wouldn't be expected that the applicant produces a full definition of either entropy or enthalpy, just that they have a qualitative understanding of what each term represents for a system.

A poor applicant fails to recall what entropy and enthalpy represent, or that they are combined in the equation for Gibbs energy. Both of these things should be second nature to applicants as they will have applied them throughout their time in higher education.

Q33: How do glow sticks work?

This question is designed to get the applicant to think outside the box, whilst applying a knowledge of Chemistry. It doesn't test knowledge of any specific topics but could be used to explore a number of different things by the interviewer. Expect to be guided by the interviewer and be curious throughout. For this question, start by answering the question in a basic sense. **A good applicant** explains that prior to use, glow sticks are dull in colour but when bent by the user, a crack is usually heard and then they glow i.e., the glow sticks produce visible light. If the applicant has not encountered a glow stick before, the interviewer may well produce one and demonstrate these facts.

The applicant should then explore this in more detail:
- The cracking noise suggests that the bending breaks something within the glowstick,
- Glowing is likely to be produced by a chemical reaction.
- Given that cracking noise precedes glowing, whatever breaks within the glow stick must lead to the reaction of two chemicals that are previously separate.

The glow stick must work by mixing two reagents, which are initially separate, but become mixed by bending the glowstick. The reaction between these two reagents produces visible light.

The interviewer will then explore how the reaction produces visible light:
- If light is produced then electrons in the glow stick must be losing energy, i.e. moving down energy levels, and releasing photons whose wavelength corresponds to the energy gap between those energy levels.
- These transitions take place within a fluorescent dye found inside the glow stick:
  ○ Firstly, a reaction must take place between two reagents within the glow stick. Hydrogen peroxide and a phenyl oxalate ester (diphenyl oxalate) are typical reagents. Prior to bending, the hydrogen peroxide is in a glass vial and the diphenyl oxalate is outside. This glass vial breaks when the glowstick is bent.

- One of the products of this reaction decomposes, releasing energy. This energy is absorbed by the fluorescent dye.
- The energy promotes electrons in the fluorescent dye to higher energy levels, and when they subsequently fall down, they release this energy in the form of photons (i.e. visible light).
- The colour of light emitted depends on the chemical structure of the dye and hence dyes with different structures give glowsticks with different colours.

The more precise details of this process might be explored by the interviewer, for example: exactly which products decompose and why, or the chemistry of the initial reaction. However, the main steps are given above.

A poor applicant tries to jump ahead and guess how a glowstick might work without thinking carefully about the specifics. For example, the applicant might assume that the light is released by de-excitation of electrons (which is correct) but suggest an incorrect reason for this de-excitation. For example, that the energy for de-excitation is provided by the bending of the glowstick. Equally, the applicant might know exactly how they work and jump to the end, and miss out key details and the chemistry behind the answer. Either is undesirable, as the interviewer wants to see your thought processes, not whether you know the answer.

Q34: Why do we prefer our meals warm?

This is a broad question, designed to surprise the applicant and make them think. The key with a question like this is to start from basics and work your way through the answer logically. Remember to focus on the chemistry as much as possible. For this question, start by explaining how taste works.

A good applicant starts by explaining that taste is a component of experience. More precisely, it is produced when our tastebuds interact with chemicals in our food. Hence, it is the chemical makeup of the food we eat that determines the experience we have while eating it. Our mind produces a certain experience with sweet foods – such as cake and chocolate – when the tastebuds interact with a set of molecules called sugars. Equally, when we consume acidic foods – lemons or tartar sauce – we experience *sourness*, which is another type of taste. All in all, there are 5 components to taste – sweet, sour, bitter, savoury, and salty – all produced by foods with a different chemistry.

When food is cooked, chemical reactions occur and change the chemical composition of food and hence how it interacts with our taste buds. These chemical changes make the nutrients and energy in our food more accessible and therefore less time and energy are wasted looking for food (we get the nutrients and energy we need from less). Our brains have evolved to produce a more pleasant reaction when we taste hot food compared to cold food, because hot food provides an evolutionary advantage as hot food allows much more energy to be consumed in a shorter time. Hence food tastes different when cooked due to chemical reactions that occur during cooking, and tastes more pleasant because our brains have evolved to produce a more pleasant experience when it is eaten.

The interviewer might move on from this to examine the chemistry involved at different stages more closely:

- Chemical changes occur including the conversion of collagen to gelatin and starches turn stiff and crunchy.
- Physical changes also occur such as moisture evaporating and fats melting.
- Both chemical and physical changes alter the texture of our food, often making it easier to break down and digest.
- Chemical reactions occur throughout the digestive system and these are made easier by the chemical changes occuring in food.
- The experience produced is mediated by chemicals in the brain called neurotransmitters that produce (in the case of hot food) a more pleasant experience.

The applicant would not be expected to know any of these bullet points, but merely to engage in the discussion which the interviewer prompts with these points – be curious!

A poor applicant fails to explore taste as a component of experience and to recognise that it is fundamentally chemical in nature. Even if this is recognised, they might fail to engage in the subsequent discussion. As mentioned above, this is a very broad question and one to which the applicant would not be expected to know the answer (at least not in full). However, the important aspects are to start from the basics of taste and use your problem-solving skills to explore the question further with the interviewer.

Q35: Why do we use water as a solvent?

This is another broad question, and tests the applicant's knowledge of the chemistry of dissolution and their willingness to scrutinise the question they are being asked. For this question, begin by exploring the chemistry of dissolution.

A good applicant states the definitions of solute, solvent, and solution:
- Solute is the substance being dissolved.
- Solvent is the substance in which the solute is dissolved.
- A solution is the combination of a solvent and a solute in a homogenous phase.

The applicant may also highlight that the distinction between solute and solvent is that the solute is always in smaller quantity than the solvent. Although this distinction is not really relevant for cases where the solute is initially a solid (as it could not be the solvent), but in cases where both solute and solvent are liquid then it is important.

A solution is diluted when the solute: solvent ratio decreased. In this example, and in other similar examples, adding water would achieve this. However, the solvent does not have to be water, for example: cooking oil (solute) is often dissolved in hexane (solvent), oils produced by the skin (solute) are commonly dissolved in acetone (solvent) and oils extracted from shale (solute) are often dissolved in benzene (solvent).

So, the answer is that we use water to dilute solutions, but only in the case where the solvent was water initially, because this will decrease the solute: solvent ratio. If the solvent was anything other than water, then the addition of water would not necessarily dilute the solution and would certainly not be the easiest way to do so. Exploring the four other options:

- If the solution is initially between a solute and solvent in which water is soluble then there are two options for what happens when water is added:
  - If the initial solute is water - e.g. water dissolved in ethanol – then the concentration of solute would increase.
  - If the initial solute is not water – e.g. methanol dissolved in ethanol - then the total solute dissolved increases, despite the concentration of the initial solute remaining unchanged. So, we would say that the concentration of the *solution* increases, whilst the concentration of the initial solute within that solution remains the same.
- If the solution is initially between a solute and a solvent in which water is not soluble, then when water is added a mixture would be formed between water and the initial solution:
  - If the original solute was insoluble in water, then its concentration would not change.
  - If the original solute was soluble in water, then its concentration would decrease, as some would become dissolved in the water.

A poor applicant suggests that all solutions are between water and a solute which is water-soluble. This is not true and will prevent engagement with the following discussion. The answer is actually simple in terms of the chemistry but requires a decent amount of thinking to be explored fully. As always, be curious!

Q36: Compare and contrast hydrochloric and phosphoric acid.

This question is testing the applicant's knowledge of acidity and the structure of common acids. To start the applicant should explore the structures and behaviour of the two acids.

$$H-Cl \; + \; H_2O \; \rightleftharpoons \; Cl^- \; + \; H_3O^+$$

$$HO-\overset{\overset{\displaystyle O}{\|}}{P}\overset{\text{\tiny ''' OH}}{\underset{\text{OH}}{}} \; + \; H_2O \; \rightleftharpoons \; {}^{-}O-\overset{\overset{\displaystyle O}{\|}}{P}\overset{\text{\tiny ''OH}}{\underset{\text{OH}}{}} \; + \; H_3O^+$$

A good applicant begins with the structures of hydrochloric acid and phosphoric acid and draws their acid dissociation equilibria.

Then compare and contrast the two acids:

- HCl is a strong acid (pKa = -7) and H_3PO_4 is a weak acid (pKa = 2).
- When HCl dissociates a H-Cl bond is broken and the negative charge is on the chlorine atom.
- When H_3PO_4 dissociates a H-O bond is broken and the negative charge is on the oxygen atom.

The interviewer might then explore why HCl is strong and H_3PO_4 is weak. The factors that contribute to the strength of an acid are:
- The strength of the bond to hydrogen.
- Stability of ion:
  - How diffuse the negative charge is.
  - How electronegative the atom/s across which the charge is spread are.

The H-Cl bond has an enthalpy of around 430 kJ mol⁻¹, whilst the O-H bond has an enthalpy of around 460 kJ mol⁻¹, so we would not expect this factor to contribute to the differences in acidity. This is especially valid considering that these enthalpies are mean averages of bond enthalpies across a range of molecules. Therefore, they do not necessarily tell us the enthalpy for the bonds in these specific molecules under these specific conditions (i.e. room temperature, atmospheric pressure and in aqueous solution).

The (Pauling) electronegativity of oxygen is 3.44 and of chlorine is 3.14, which would suggest phosphoric acid to be stronger. However, we must also consider the area across which the charge is spread also. The chloride ion is large (0.181 nm), whilst that of O^{2-} is small (0.141 nm). Additionally, the negative charge on phosphoric acid's conjugate base is spread across two oxygen atoms:

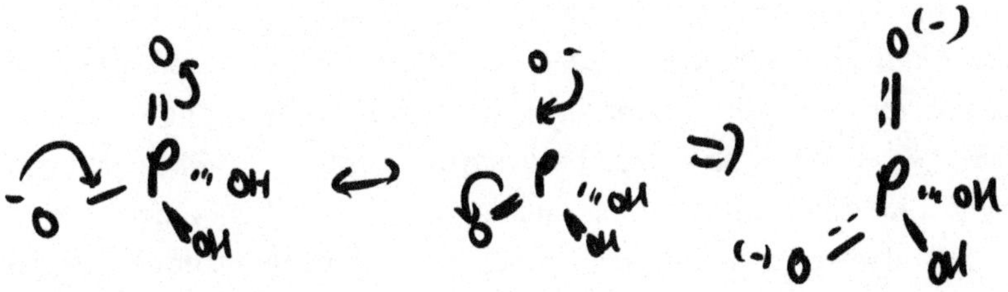

Given that the pKₐ values show HCl to be much stronger, this suggests that the large size of the chloride ion outweighs the fact that in phosphoric acid's conjugate base the charge is spread across two atoms, both of which are more electronegative than chlorine.

This latter discussion about the factors affecting pKₐ would be tackled with the interviewer and applicants would not be expected to know the specifics without prompts and guidance.

A poor applicant does not know the structures of HCl or H_3PO_4 and fails to compare and contrast the two acids. The applicant may also fail to engage in the higher-level discussion about the factors influencing acidity. This discussion is key to comparing and contrasting the two acids and includes some really interesting elements of acid-base theory which the applicant isn't likely to be familiar with.

Q37: What makes vanadium special?

This is another open question, and one to which there is not necessarily a right answer. The key here is to demonstrate any knowledge you have about vanadium, as well as closely related chemistry, and to be prepared for discussions beyond what you know already.

A good applicant begins by mentioning that vanadium is unique because it has 23 protons. No other element has 23 protons, by definition. Vanadium is also unique in that, in a neutral state, it has 23 electrons, each of which is in an electrostatic environment unique to an atom of vanadium. These are statements which could be made about *any* element – but which also provide the insight that the chemistry of vanadium will also be unique. No other element has electrons in the environments that vanadium does, and so the chemical reactions of vanadium, although they may show similarities to other elements, will be unique.

The applicant can then discuss more broad elements of vanadium's chemistry. For example:

- Vanadium is a transition metal and has one or more stable ions with an incomplete d-shell. It also exhibits colourful complexes, variable oxidation states and can be used as a catalyst.
- Vanadium is a metal and is likely to be shiny, malleable, ductile, a good conductor of heat and electricity and to have high melting and boiling points.

More specific examples could include:

- Vanadium (V) oxide is used as catalyst in the contact process for producing sulfur trioxide:

$$SO_2 + V_2O_5 \rightsquigarrow SO_3 + V_2O_4$$

$$V_2O_4 + \tfrac{1}{2}O_2 \rightarrow V_2O_5$$

$$i.e \quad SO_2 + \tfrac{1}{2}O_2 \xrightarrow{V_2O_5} SO_3 \quad overall$$

- Vanadium's variable oxidation states are showcased in the following sequence (in which zinc can be used as the reducing agent, or acid as an oxidising agent if we want to go in the reverse direction):

$$VO_2^+ \rightarrow VO^{2+} \rightarrow \left[V(H_2O)_6\right]^{3+} \rightarrow \left[V(H_2O)_6\right]^{2+}$$
$$(V) \qquad (IV) \qquad (III) \qquad (II)$$

A poor applicant fails to recognise the properties that make vanadium, and indeed any element, unique. They may also miss specific elements of vanadium's chemistry, which the applicant should be familiar with from school.

Q38: Where is the line between chemistry and physics?

This is a broad question, designed to test your lateral thinking skills as well as your knowledge of physics and chemistry. There's not necessarily a right answer, but the interviewer is looking to confirm the applicant knows what chemistry and physics entail, and the boundary between the sciences. As usual, engaging in the process in a logical way is key.

A good applicant starts by recognising that chemistry is the study of elements, how they bond to one another and how those bonds may change in chemical reactions. Chemistry encompasses the following: the structure of atoms to the structure of giant molecular structures and from kinetics to thermodynamics. Physics, meanwhile, studies the laws of nature: from Newton's laws of motion to Boyle's law for gases, from the behaviour of the strong nuclear force to the nature of electrostatic interactions. Here the applicant might notice elements of crossover:

- The nature of electrostatic interactions governs the electronic energy levels present in atoms.
- The nature of the strong nuclear force has implications for the structure of nuclei (and hence atoms).

Given that the laws of nature must, ultimately, control everything that happens, they must explain everything that happens in chemistry. That is not to say that all areas of physics are relevant for chemists – Newton's laws, for example, have limited applications in chemistry. But there are a set of physical laws, discovered by physicists, which must govern all that happens in chemistry.

Here, an example is illustrative, and applicants could choose from a range such as nuclear physics, quantum physics, solid-state physics, materials science etc. We will tackle Quantum physics here.

Physicists have an area of study concerned with the nature of matter on the smallest scales – quantum physics. This encompasses how the particles in nuclei interact with one another, how electrons interact with one another and with nuclei etc. The laws that govern these processes are therefore vital knowledge for understanding the structure of atoms and therefore how they will combine to form simple molecules, giant molecules, ionic lattices etc. For physicists, the focus is the bigger picture – what is the ultimate nature of these interactions? But chemists are interested in exactly how these laws influence the structure of specific substances and the development of specific reactions. Physicists do not concern themselves with organic functional groups, or the mechanism of nucleophilic substitution, despite the fact that both of these things are derived from the laws of quantum physics in some sense.

Overall, physicists and chemists study many of the same things, but in different ways. Physicists are more abstract, while chemists are more practical. Physicists care about general principles, whilst chemists are concerned with specific examples. Both have an important role to play.

The latter part of this discussion would likely be prompted by the interviewer, as no applicant would be expected to have already come to this conclusion. The most important thing is to think carefully about differences between the sciences, and show what you know about both and provide specific and clear examples.

A poor applicant fails to recognise the characteristics of chemistry and physics, as without this information it will be hard to work towards the point at which the subjects intersect. The applicant may also fail to engage properly with the discussion.

Q39: How would you turn endothermic reaction into an exothermic one?

This question is testing the applicant's knowledge of thermodynamics. To start, the applicant should explore the nature of an endothermic reaction.

A good applicant: Starts by defining an endothermic reaction as one in which the enthalpy change is positive. For a system at constant pressure and temperature, this is identical to the statement that heat is absorbed by the system during an endothermic reaction. Then the applicant moves on to discuss whether the nature of a given reaction could be changed, using an example such as the dissolution of salt in water:

$$NaCl_{(s)} \longrightarrow Na^+_{(aq)} + Cl^-_{(aq)} \quad \Delta H < 0$$

The applicant might reason that however this process is completed, the initial and final states are the same. The enthalpy of the initial and final states would therefore be the same and so the enthalpy change for the reaction must be the same regardless of how the reaction is carried out. Other example reactions could also be used here to explain the point made.

Another way this conclusion could be reached is by a knowledge of thermodynamic cycles. Often, to calculate bond enthalpies or lattice energies, we used a thermodynamic cycle such as the Born-Haber cycle. The whole premise of this method is that the enthalpy change for a reaction is identical regardless of the route taken. An example might be drawn:

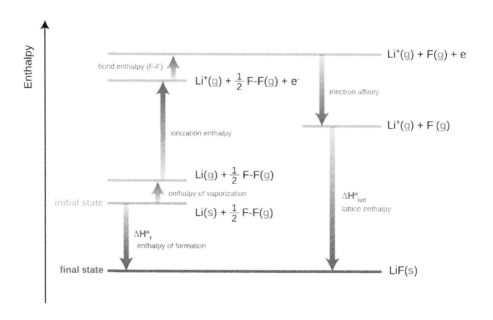

Hence the answer is no, not only can an endothermic reaction not be made exothermic, but the enthalpy change for a given reaction cannot be changed in any way. The interviewer might lead the discussion from this point by comparing state and path functions. Enthalpy is a state function because it depends only on the physical state of the system, not how that state was reached. However, the heat energy supplied is a path function because it depends on the path taken between two states. As mentioned above, the enthalpy change and heat supplied are equal *only in the case where pressure and temperature are constant*, hence in any other case the heat supplied might be different despite the enthalpy change being the same for a given reaction.

A poor applicant suggests that an endothermic reaction could be made exothermic, or that the enthalpy change for a reaction might be different depending on the path taken. This is basic thermodynamic knowledge and should be second nature to applicants at this level.

READING LISTS

The obvious way to prepare for any Oxbridge interview is to **read widely**. This is important so that you can mention books and interests in your personal statement. It is also important because it means that you will be able to draw upon a greater number and variety of ideas for your interview.

- **Make a record** of the book, who wrote it, when they wrote it, and summarise the argument. This means that you have some details about your research in the days before the interview.

- Reading is a passive exercise. To make it genuinely meaningful, you should **engage with the text**. Summarise the argument. Ask yourself questions like how is the writer arguing? Is it a compelling viewpoint?

- **Quality over quantity**. This is not a race as to how many books you can read in a short period of time. It is instead a test of your ability to critically analyse and synthesise information from a text – something you'll be doing on a daily basis at university.

BIOLOGY & MEDICINE

- *Bad Pharma*: Ben Goldacre
- *Trust me I'm a Junior Doctor*: Max Pemberton
- *The Selfish Gene*: Richard Dawkins
- *Genome*: Matt Ridley
- *The Single Helix*: Steve Jones
- Nature via Nurture: Matt Ridley
- *Bully for Brontosaurus*: Stephen Jay Gould
- *The Extended Phenotype*: Richard Dawkins

PSYCHOLOGY

- *The Man who Mistook his Wife for a Hat:* Oliver Sacks
- *How the Mind Works:* Steven Pinker
- *Predictably Irrational:* Dan Ariely
- *Thinking, Fast and Slow:* Daniel Kahneman

CHEMISTRY

- *The Disappearing Spoon:* Sam Kean
- *Uncle Tungsten:* Oliver Sacks
- *A Short history of Nearly Everything:* Bill Bryson
- *Reactions- The Private Life of Atoms:* Peter Atkins

FINAL ADVICE

BEFORE YOUR INTERVIEW

- Make sure you understand your curriculum; your interview will most likely use material from your school courses as a starting point.

- Remind yourself of the selection criteria for your subject.

- Read around your subject in scientific articles and books, visit museums, watch documentaries, anything which broadens your knowledge of your favourite topics while demonstrating your passion for your subject. They may ask you at the interview which articles you've read recently to check you are engaged with the subject. Scientists should try New Scientist's online articles to start you off; TED talks are also a great way to be quickly briefed on cutting-edge research, and it's more likely you will remember the name of the researcher, etc.

- Practice common questions or sample questions – this is better done with a teacher or someone you are less familiar with or who is an experienced interviewer.

- Make up your own questions throughout your day: Why is that flower shaped like that? Why is that bird red-breasted? Why does my dog like to fetch sticks? What did I mean when I said that man wasn't 'normal', and is this the criteria everyone uses? How do I know I see the same colours as others?

- Re-read your personal statement and any coursework you are providing. Anticipate questions that may arise from these and prepare them in advance.

- Read and do anything you've said you've done in your application – they may ask you about it at the interview!

- Check your interview specifications – what type of interviews you will have for which subjects, how many there will be, where, when, and with whom they will be so there are no surprises.

ON THE DAY OF YOUR INTERVIEW

- Get a good night's sleep before the big day.

- If you are travelling from far away, try to arrive the night before so that you're fresh in the morning. Getting up early in the morning and travelling far could tire you out and you might be less focused whilst being interviewed. Many colleges will provide you accommodation if you're travelling from a certain distance away.

- Take a shower in the morning and dress to your comfort, though you don't want to give a sloppy first impression – most opt for smart/casual

- Get there early so you aren't late or stressed out before it even starts.

- Smile at everyone and be polite.

- Don't worry about other candidates; be nice of course, but you are there for you, and their impressions of how their interviews went have nothing to do with what the interviewers thought or how yours will go.

- It's OK to be nervous – they know you're nervous and understand, but try to move past it and be in the moment to get the most out of the experience.

- Don't be discouraged if it feels like one interview didn't go well – you may have shown the interviewers exactly what they wanted to see, even if it wasn't what you wanted to see.

- Have a cuppa and relax, there's nothing you can do now but be yourself.

THE MOST IMPORTANT ADVICE...

- ❖ Explain your thought processes as much as possible – it doesn't matter if you're wrong. *It really is the journey; not the destination that matters.*

- ❖ Interviewers aren't interested in *what you know*. Instead, they are more interested in *what you can do* with what you already know.

✗ **DON'T** be quiet – even if you can't answer a question. How you approach the question could show the interviewer what they want to see.

✗ **DON'T** rely on the interviewer to guide you every step of the way.

✗ **DON'T** ever, ever, ever give up.

✗ **DON'T** be arrogant or rigid –you are bound to get things wrong, just accept them and move on.

✗ **DON'T** expect to know all the answers; this is different than school, you aren't expected to know the answer to everything – you are using your knowledge as a foundation for original thoughts and applications under the guidance of your interviewer.

✗ **DON'T** think you will remember everything you did/wrote without revising.

✗ **DON'T** be afraid to point out flaws in your own ideas – scientists need to be self-critical, and the interviewer has already noticed your mistakes!

✗ **DON'T** be defensive, especially if the interviewer is hinting that your idea may be on the wrong path – the interviewer is the expert!

✗ **DON'T** get hung up on a question for too long.

✗ **DON'T** rehearse scripted answers to be regurgitated.

✗ **DON'T** answer the question you wanted them to ask.

✗ **DON'T** lie about things you have read/done (and if you already lied in your personal statement, then read/do them before the interview!).

✓ **DO** speak freely about what you are thinking and ask for clarifications.

✓ **DO** take suggestions and listen for pointers from your interviewer.

✓ **DO** try your best to get to the answer.

✓ **DO** have confidence in yourself and the abilities that got you this far

✓ **DO** be prepared to discuss the ideas and problems in your work.

✓ **DO** make many suggestions and have many ideas.

✓ **DO** show intellectual flexibility by taking suggestions from the interviewer.

✓ **DO** take your time in answering to ensure your words come out right.

✓ **DO** research your interviewers so that you know their basic research interests. Then ensure you understand the basics of their work (no need to go into detail with this).

✓ **DO** prepare your answers to common questions.

✓ **DO** answer the question that the interviewer has asked – not the one you want them to!

✓ **DO** practice interviews with family or teachers – even easy questions may be harder to articulate out loud and on the spot to a stranger.

✓ **DO** think about strengths/experiences you may wish to highlight.

✓ **DO** visit www.uniadmissions.co.uk/example-interviews to see mock interviews in your subject. This will allow you to understand the differences between good and bad candidates.

AFTERWORD

Remember that the route to success is your approach and practice. Don't fall into the trap that *"you can't prepare for Oxbridge interviews"*– this could not be further from the truth. With targeted preparation and focused reading, you can dramatically boost your chances of getting that dream offer.

Work hard, never give up, and do yourself justice.

Good luck!

This book is dedicated to my grandparents – thank you for your wisdom, kindness, and endless amounts of love.

Acknowledgements

I would like to express my gratitude to the many people who helped make this book possible. I would like to thank *Dr. Ranjna Garg* for suggesting that I take on this mammoth task and providing invaluable feedback. I am also grateful for the 30 Oxbridge tutors for their specialist input and advice. Last, but by no means least; I am thankful to *David Salt* for his practical advice and willingness to discuss my ideas- regardless of whether it was 4 AM or 4 PM.

About Us

We currently publish over 100 titles across a range of subject areas – covering specialised admissions tests, examination techniques, personal statement guides, plus everything else you need to improve your chances of getting on to competitive courses such as medicine and law, as well as into universities such as Oxford and Cambridge.

Outside of publishing we also operate a highly successful tuition division, called UniAdmissions. This company was founded in 2013 by Dr Rohan Agarwal and Dr David Salt, both Cambridge Medical graduates with several years of tutoring experience. Since then, every year, hundreds of applicants and schools work with us on our programmes. Through the programmes we offer, we deliver expert tuition, exclusive course places, online courses, best-selling textbooks and much more.

With a team of over 1,000 Oxbridge tutors and a proven track record, UniAdmissions have quickly become the UK's number one admissions company.

Visit and engage with us at:

Website (UniAdmissions): www.uniadmissions.co.uk
Facebook: www.facebook.com/uniadmissionsuk

Printed in Great Britain
by Amazon

11664820R00231